EGG FREEZING
—— IN THE ——
21ST CENTURY

A Global Perspective

Other Titles by the Editor

Fertility and Infertility For Dummies

EGG FREEZING
—— IN THE ——
21ST CENTURY

A Global Perspective

Foreword by **Roy Homburg**

Editor

Gillian Lockwood
CARE Fertility Tamworth, UK

W⊖ World Scientific

NEW JERSEY · LONDON · SINGAPORE · BEIJING · SHANGHAI · HONG KONG · TAIPEI · CHENNAI · TOKYO

Published by

World Scientific Publishing Co. Pte. Ltd.

5 Toh Tuck Link, Singapore 596224

USA office: 27 Warren Street, Suite 401-402, Hackensack, NJ 07601

UK office: 57 Shelton Street, Covent Garden, London WC2H 9HE

Library of Congress Cataloging-in-Publication Data

Names: Lockwood, Gillian, editor.

Title: Egg freezing in the 21st century : a global perspective / editor,
   Gillian Lockwood ; foreword by Roy Homburg.

Other titles: Egg freezing in the twenty-first century

Description: New Jersey : World Scientific, [2024] | Includes bibliographical references and index.

Identifiers: LCCN 2023052491 | ISBN 9789811253003 (hardcover) |
   ISBN 9789811253010 (ebook for institution) | ISBN 9789811253027 (ebook for individuals)

Subjects: MESH: Fertility Preservation--methods | Oocyte Donation | Infertility, Female--therapy

Classification: LCC RG201 | NLM WQ 208 | DDC 618.1/78--dc23/eng/20240301

LC record available at https://lccn.loc.gov/2023052491

British Library Cataloguing-in-Publication Data

A catalogue record for this book is available from the British Library.

For any available supplementary material, please visit
https://www.worldscientific.com/worldscibooks/10.1142/12745#t=suppl

Desk Editor: Shaun Tan Yi Jie

Typeset by Stallion Press
Email: enquiries@stallionpress.com

Foreword

Roy Homburg

Two apparently diametrically opposed issues have lately been talking points of the scientific community: global warming and egg freezing. While the first has produced little in the way of international cooperation and tangible progress, the latest research and practical application of egg vitrification is proving a real advance and benefit in the world of reproductive medicine.

In this volume, Gillian Lockwood has gathered leading embryologists, scientists, clinicians and ethicists to describe their research and views on every aspect of egg freezing. None could be better equipped than Dr Lockwood to edit this volume as she has a background in ethics and public policy and was the first to produce a 'frozen egg' baby in the UK in 2002. Her 20 years of experience in the field have enabled her to reach out to international colleagues to contribute to this book.

It is so-called "social" egg freezing that has mainly caught public attention due to the enticing prospect of the ability to prolong the fertile age allowing career women and those presently without a partner to delay their childbearing aspirations. Despite vast media coverage and the taking up of the idea by very large companies offering their female workers free access to the procedure in order to keep them at work, few realise that this is no cast-iron guarantee for success. Chapters in this book offer the correct approach to the subject, setting out the conditions needed for success, up-to-date success rates and even the ethical issues relating to ownership, disposal and donation of cryopreserved eggs. The true impact of social egg freezing is yet to play out so the solid base provided by this book is of immense importance.

Fertility preservation, rather than fertility extension, has presented a quite different challenge. In the past, the devastation of a pronounced life-threatening diagnosis concentrated the minds of young women on how to endure the punishing treatment and how to cope with the predicted life expectancy. The loss of fertility potential induced by chemotherapy and radiation was of secondary importance to survival. This picture has changed quite dramatically as the prognosis following treatment has improved markedly and egg vitrification is widely available. Most oncologists are now fully aware of the possibilities of the preservation of fertility by egg freezing, which can now be offered to most of these patients before starting cancer treatment. Decisions must be speedily taken as regards timing and the possibilities of collecting a suitable number of eggs in the time available.

While I have only referred to egg freezing, there are proven alternatives to achieve the same aims. One of these is the freezing of the ovarian cortex which contains a vast number of primordial follicles and which can be thawed and implanted at various sites, usually in the pelvis, and has been proven capable of engendering a pregnancy. This method has also been controversially touted as a way to delay the onset of menopause, a subject still in its infancy.

The 'headliners' above belie the enormous amount of research that has gone into their establishment. The history and development of oocyte cryopreservation are described fittingly in the first chapter of this book and bear witness to what has been achieved so far. The latest research has outlined methodologies for optimising laboratory performance and many technical developments in oocyte vitrification. Clinicians have also had to find optimal management strategies for patents involved in oocyte-freezing protocols, the most suitable ovarian stimulation and the optimal protocol for frozen/thawed blastocyst transfer for example. Many of these have, of course, to be adapted to individual needs and these are extensively covered in this volume.

The first inkling of the possibilities of egg freezing came from Chen in the Far East in 1986. Since then, progress has been enormous and the innovations have been applied worldwide. It is further proof that science has no borders and the global nature of our profession, whether clinicians, embryologists, scientists, ethicists or counsellors working for a common goal, bears witness to this. This is reflected not only in the title of this book referring to 'A Global Perspective' but in the truly international array of contributors.

Gillian Lockwood is to be congratulated in gathering the top experts in the field from all corners of the globe and producing a book which will be of immense value and a fund of knowledge for all concerned in this fascinating topic.

About the Editor

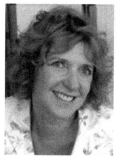

Dr Gillian M Lockwood was most recently Medical Director at CARE Fertility Tamworth, UK, before her retirement. She is a Fellow of the Royal College of Obstetrics and Gynaecology, and holds a PhD from the University of Oxford. She was previously Medical Director for 20 years at Midland Fertility which produced the UK's first 'frozen egg' baby in 2002. She has published more than 50 papers on all aspects of fertility, and co-authored the book *Fertility & Infertility for Dummies*.

Dr Lockwood lectures widely on the ethics and economics of 'social' egg freezing. She was previously Chair of the British Fertility Society Ethics Sub-Committee, Vice Chair of the RCOG Ethics Committee, and Special Advisor to the UK Parliament Select Committee on Science and Technology which undertook a review of the Human Fertilisation and Embryology Act.

About the Contributors

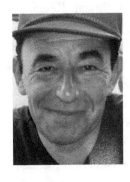

Professor Roy Homburg, MBBS, FRCOG *ad eundem*, has held posts as Professor of Obstetrics and Gynaecology at Tel Aviv University, Israel, Professor of Reproductive Medicine at VU University Medical Centre, The Netherlands, at Queen Mary University of London, UK and at Hewitt Fertility Centre, UK. He has published 320 articles/chapters in books and has written/edited 13 books. He has been invited to lecture worldwide frequently and has won prizes for research from the British Fertility Society (BFS), the American Society for Reproductive Medicine (ASRM), the European Society of Human Reproduction and Embryology (ESHRE) and the Israel Fertility Society. He has served as Associate Editor for *Human Reproduction* and *Human Reproduction Update*, and Section Editor for *Reproductive Biology and Endocrinology*. He was the International Adviser to the SIG Reproductive Endocrinology of ESHRE, and is the Principal

Coordinator of Reproductive Endocrinology and Infertility of the International Society for In Vitro Fertilization.

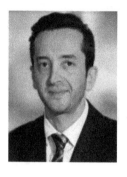

Dr Georgios Petsas, MD, PhD, is the Medical Director at Care Fertility Sheffield, UK. He graduated from the University of Crete Medical School, Greece, in 2003 and completed his specialist training in Obstetrics and Gynaecology in the University Hospital of Heraklion, Greece. In 2013 he completed his PhD on the role of hypothalamic neuropeptides in early embryo implantation and in the pathophysiology of diseases with defective placentation at the University of Crete Medical School. Soon after, he went on to complete a Clinical Research Fellowship in the UK where he developed a special interest in fertility preservation.

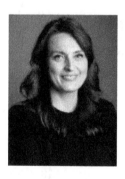

Associate Professor Evrim Ünsal, PhD, started her professional career as an Embryologist in 1997 and received her PhD from the Institute of Biotechnology, Ankara University, Turkey in 2007. She received the title of Associate Professor in 2016 at the Yüksek İhtisas University in Turkey and has worked as the Director of the Mikrogen Genetic Diagnostic Laboratory where she continued her studies on pre-implantation genetic testing, carrier screening and next-generation sequencing-based comprehensive genetic tests. She served on the Board of the Clinical Embryology Society for 12 years, and organised many hands-on workshops and training programs. As the Special Interest Group Coordinator of the Turkish Society of Reproductive Medicine, she has organised many events concerning screening for rare diseases, and is currently working as an Associate Research Scientist at the Yale University Fertility Clinic, USA.

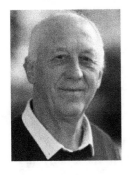

Professor Claus Yding Andersen, MSc, DMSc, is Professor Emeritus of Human Reproductive Physiology at the Faculty of Health and Medical Sciences, University of Copenhagen, Denmark. He has headed a national program on cryopreservation of human ovarian and testicular tissue and is considered one of the pioneers in this field. His major research contributions are ovarian endocrinology, oocyte maturation, cryopreservation of gonadal tissue, and development of new principles for ovarian stimulation, including the agonist trigger and novel approaches to luteal phase support. He has published more than 460 papers (H-index: 91; >27,000 citations) and is Chief Editor on the Reproduction section of *Frontiers in Endocrinology* (impact factor 5.2).

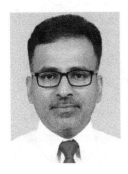

Dr Abey Eapen, MD, PhD, graduated in Medicine from the University of Calicut, India. He underwent his basic training in Obstetrics and Gynaecology and further specialist training in Reproductive Medicine in the UK. He successfully completed a PhD in Reproductive Medicine from the University of Birmingham, UK and a Fellowship in Reproductive Immunology from the American Society of Reproductive Immunology, USA. Currently, he is employed as a Clinical Associate Professor in the Division of Reproductive Endocrinology and Infertility at the University of Iowa Hospitals and Clinics, USA. His research interests include recurrent pregnancy loss and recurrent implantation failure.

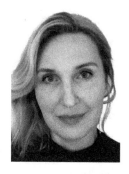

Dr Karolina Palinska-Rudzka, MRCOG, MD, graduated from the Medical University of Warsaw, Poland and later pursued her Specialty Training in Obstetrics and Gynaecology in the West Midlands, UK. Her academic pursuits led her to complete an MD degree at the University of Warwick, UK. During this time, she led a project investigating ovarian reserve in young women with cancer undergoing gonadotoxic therapy, under the supervision of Dr Gillian Lockwood and Professor Geraldine Hartshorne. This research has been presented both nationally and internationally. She recently completed her Subspecialty Training in Reproductive Medicine and is currently employed at the Department of Reproductive Medicine in St. Mary's Hospital, UK.

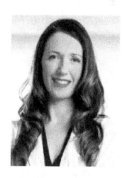

Dr Anabel Salazar Vera, MD, has been Gynaecologist Specialist in Reproductive Medicine at IVIRMA Global since 2007 and Medical Director of the IVI Málaga clinic since 2013. She qualified in Medicine and Surgery from the University of Cádiz, Spain, in 2002 and was in the specialty of Obstetrics and Gynaecology at the Juan Ramón Jiménez Hospital in Spain, 2003–2007.

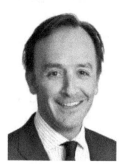

Professor Juan García-Velasco, MD, PhD, is Chief Scientific Officer of IVIRMA Global and Director of IVIRMA Madrid. He is also Professor of Obstetrics and Gynaecology at Rey Juan Carlos University, Spain, where he is Director of the Master's Degree Programme in Human Reproduction. His main research interests have been in *in vitro* fertilisation and endometriosis. He is the Principal Investigator of projects funded by the Ministry of Education and Ministry of Health in Spain, and has received awards from the Spanish Fertility Society, Spanish Society of Obstetrics and Gynaecology, and ESHRE. He has published over 200 peer-reviewed articles, 30 book chapters and 6 books on human reproduction, endometriosis and hypo- and hyper-ovarian stimulation response. He is the co-Editor-in-Chief of *Reproductive Biomedicine Online*.

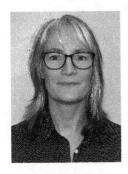

Rachel Smith, BSc, is a registered clinical scientist and embryologist and after 18 years of being Laboratory Manager at CARE Sheffield, UK, she expanded her role to a central and corporate leadership position. She is currently Embryology Innovation and Artificial Intelligence Lead. The role focuses on new technology, automation and research, driving improvements in patient success rates, laboratory efficiencies and consistency across the group. In addition, she holds the Person Responsible position which she has undertaken for 15 years at CARE Sheffield and continues to provide support in the laboratory when required.

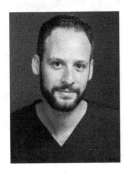

Dr Dan Nayot, BSc, MD, FRCSC, is a practicing Reproductive Endocrinologist & Infertility (REI) Specialist at The Reproductive Care Centre in Canada and Medical Director at The Fertility Partners, a North American network of *in vitro* fertilisation clinics. He is also the Co-Founder and Chief Medical Officer at Future Fertility Inc. He completed his BSc in Mathematics at the University of Toronto, Canada, MD at the

University of Western Ontario, Canada, Master of Clinical Epidemiology at Harvard University, USA, FRCSC in Obstetrics and Gynaecology at the University of Toronto, and REI Fellowship at McGill University, Canada. He is committed to innovation and data-driven research to optimise the patient experience and expand access to fertility care.

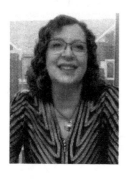

Professor Marcia C Inhorn, PhD, MPH, is the William K. Lanman Jr. Professor of Anthropology and International Affairs at Yale University, USA where she serves as Chair of the Council on Middle East Studies. A medical anthropologist specializing in Middle Eastern gender, religion, and reproductive health issues, she has conducted research on the social impact of infertility and assisted reproductive technologies in Egypt, Lebanon, the United Arab Emirates, and Arab America over the past 35 years. She is the author of six books on the subject, including *America's Arab Refugees: Vulnerability and Health on the Margins* (Stanford University Press, 2018). She has recently published her seventh book called *Motherhood on Ice: The Mating Gap and Why Women Freeze Their Eggs,* based on a US National Science Foundation-funded study of 150 American women who undertook egg freezing, primarily because of partnership problems.

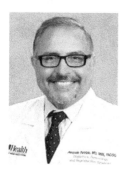

Professor Pasquale Patrizio, MD, MBE, HCLD, FACOG, is Professor of Obstetrics/Gynaecology and Chief, Division of Reproductive Endocrinology and Infertility, at the Miller School of Medicine, University of Miami, USA. He is a section editor for the *American Journal of Obstetrics and Gynaecology* and *Reproductive*

Biomedicine Online, and is editorial board member for the *Journal of Assisted Reproduction and Genetics*. In 2007, he co-founded the International Society for Fertility Preservation and served as president between 2015–2017. He has authored 9 books, 625 scientific papers (91 book chapters, 238 peer-reviewed publications and 296 published abstracts) and holds 2 issued patents. He is Honorary Member of the Italian Society of Fertility and Sterility, Fellow of the International Academy of Human Reproduction, and has received many prizes and paper awards from both ASRM and ESHRE.

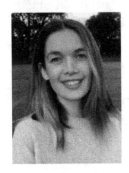

Dr Molly Johnston, PhD, is a Research Fellow at the Monash Bioethics Centre, Monash University, Australia. She was awarded her PhD from Monash University in 2021. She has a background in reproductive science but her current research falls within the intersection between social science, bioethics, and regulation. Her research interests are the ethical, social, and regulatory issues raised by human reproductive technologies, in particular assisted reproduction and prenatal genetic testing.

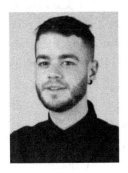

Dr Michiel De Proost, PhD, is a postdoctoral researcher at the Department of Philosophy and Moral Sciences at Ghent University, Belgium and is affiliated with the Bioethics Institute Ghent and the METAMEDICA consortium. His academic research focuses on feminist bioethics, disruptive technologies in medicine, and practices of responsibility.

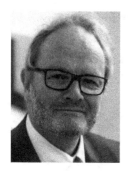

Professor Nick Macklon, DPhil, FRCOG, is Group Medical Director of London Women's Clinic, London Sperm Bank and London Egg Bank. Prior to this he held Departmental Chair positions and full professorships at the Universities of Utrecht, Southampton and Copenhagen, where he is a Visiting Professor. His widely published research has received international award recognition and he has supervised over 25 PhD projects to completion. A former member of the ESHRE Executive Committee, he has acted as Associate Editor for *Human Reproduction* and *Human Reproduction Update*, and was recently appointed co-Chief Editor of *Reproductive BioMedicine Online.*

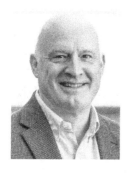

Professor Alan Pacey, PhD, FRCOG *ad eundem*, MBE, recently joined the University of Manchester, UK where he is the Deputy Vice President and Deputy Dean of the Faculty of Biology, Medicine and Health. He is also Professor of Andrology and has published over 200 research papers, book chapters and review articles. He is a former Secretary (2005–2010) and Chairman (2012–2015) of BFS and former Editor-in-Chief of the BFS journal *Human Fertility* (2015–2022). In addition, he is an accomplished science communicator and broadcaster. Recent television programmes include Me, My Brother and our Balls (2020), Alex Jones: Fertility & Me (2016), Britain's Secret Code Breaker (2011), Donor Unknown (2011), The Great Sperm Race (2009), The Truth About Food (2007), Make me a Baby (2007) and Lab Rats (2004). Awards include a Fellowship *ad eundem* of the Royal College of Obstetricians and Gynaecologists (2014) in recognition of contributions to the speciality and wellbeing of women, an MBE from Her Majesty Queen Elizabeth II for services to reproductive medicine (2016), and Honorary (lifetime) Fellowship from BFS (2023).

https://doi.org/10.1142/9789811253010_fmatter

Contents

Foreword   v
About the Editor   viii
About the Contributors   ix

Chapter 1   Where Have All the Babies Gone?   1
             Gillian Lockwood

Chapter 2   History and Development of Oocyte
             Cryopreservation   16
             Georgios Petsas

Chapter 3   Human Oocyte Freezing Technologies: Current
             State-of-Art and Future Perspectives   31
             Evrim Ünsal

Chapter 4   Alternatives to Oocyte Cryopreservation: Ovarian
             Cortex Freezing and *In Vitro* Maturation   47
             Claus Yding Andersen

Chapter 5   Worldwide Trends in Oocyte Cryopreservation;
             Maternal and Neonatal Outcomes Following
             Oocyte Cryopreservation   66
             Abey Eapen

Chapter 6   Social Egg Freezing from a UK Perspective:
             Can it Help Keep Us Warm in the Coming
             'Demographic Winter'?   86
             Gillian Lockwood

Chapter 7   The Assessment of Ovarian Reserve Prior to
             Oocyte Freezing   107
             Karolina Palinska-Rudzka

Chapter 8   Clinical Management of Oocyte Vitrification
             Patients: Stimulation Protocols and Frozen/
             Thawed Blastocyst Transfer Protocols   122
             Anabel Salazar Vera and Juan A Garcia-Velasco

Chapter 9   The Application of Artificial Intelligence to
             Oocyte Evaluation: Methods, Scope and
             Limitations   151
             Rachel Smith and Dan Nayot

Chapter 10   Public Perceptions and Societal Attitudes versus
             Egg Freezing Realities   166
             Marcia C. Inhorn and Pasquale Patrizio

Chapter 11   Funding the Future Family: An Unsettled Moral
             Issue   186
             Molly Johnston and Michiel De Proost

Chapter 12   Egg Donation: The Future is Frozen   205
             Nick Macklon, V Pataia and K Ahuja

Chapter 13   Male Attitudes to Oocyte Cryopreservation   221
             Allan Pacey

Index   237

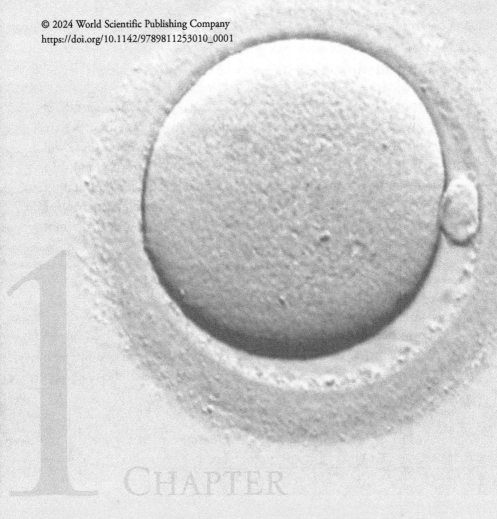

1

CHAPTER

Where Have All the
Babies Gone?

Gillian Lockwood

1.1 Introduction

There appear to be two inconsistent, yet equally worrying, narratives being advanced at present concerning the world's population. We are warned that we are 'running out' of babies (Figure 1.1) and there will be no one to care for us in our (increasing) old age nor pay our pensions, and yet, simultaneously, the world is facing a 'population explosion' (Figure 1.2) which will herald unsustainable demand for resources, resulting in environmental degradation, resource depletion, mass migration and, inevitably, worldwide conflict.

1.2 Our Expanding Planet

The world population has experienced a significant increase over the past two centuries. In 1800, the world's population was around one

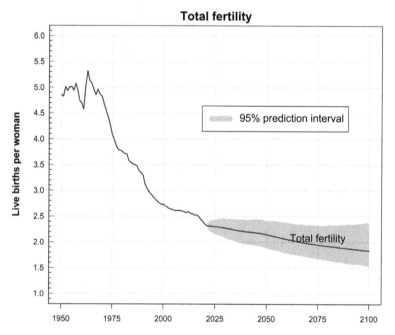

Figure 1.1   Total world fertility rate with projection. Source: United Nations.

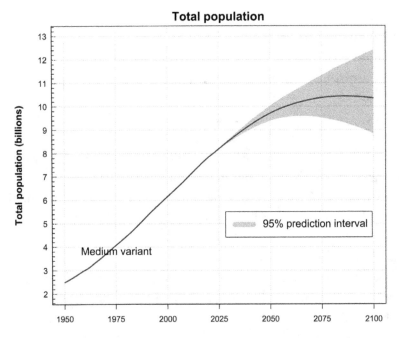

Figure 1.2   Total world population with projection. Source: United Nations.

billion people, and by the end of the 20th century, it had reached six billion. As we move further into the 21st century, the population continues to grow, and estimates suggest that it could reach 9.7 billion by 2050.

During the 19th century, the world population grew slowly. It took almost 100 years for the population to double, reaching two billion in 1927. However, the 20th century saw significant growth and the world population doubled again, reaching four billion by 1974, and then six billion by 1999. This rapid growth was fuelled by many factors, including improvements in healthcare, sanitation, and nutrition, which led to a decrease in mortality rates and an increase in life expectancy.

Other factors contributing to the population growth were the continuing industrial and agrarian revolutions, resulting in increased agricultural productivity and allowing for larger populations to be sustained on land enhanced with chemical fertilisers and worked with sophisticated machinery. Initially these factors influenced the population increases of the so-called developed world, but now most of this growth is occurring in developing countries.

However, the world population growth figures and projections disguise significant differences between continents and even between adjacent countries over the past two centuries.

In 1800, the largest continent in terms of population was Asia, with approximately 650 million people, followed by Europe with approximately 200 million people. Africa had the smallest population at this time, with just over 100 million people.

By 1950, the population of all continents had increased significantly. Asia remained the most populous continent, with around 1.4 billion people, followed by Europe with approximately 547 million people. Africa's population had doubled to approximately 228 million people.

In the 21st century, the population growth of each continent has varied. Asia remains the most populous continent, with a population of approximately 4.6 billion people in 2021. Africa is the second most populous continent, with a population of approximately 1.3 billion people. Europe's population has remained relatively stable at around 747 million people, while North America's population has increased to around 596 million people.

South America's population has also increased significantly since 1950, from approximately 167 million people to around 429 million people in 2021. Oceania's population has also grown, from around 14 million people in 1950 to around 42 million people in 2021.

The population growth rates of each continent have also varied. Africa has had the highest population growth rate, with an average annual growth rate of around 2.5% between 2010 and 2020. Asia's population growth rate has been declining over time, from an average annual growth rate of around 2.3% between 1950 and 1960 to around 0.8% between 2010 and 2020. Europe and North America have had relatively low population growth rates, with rates of around 0.2% and 0.7%, respectively, between 2010 and 2020.

Africa has the youngest population of any continent, with a median age of 19.7 years as of 2020. According to the United Nations, in 2020, approximately 20% of Africa's population was between the ages of 15 and 24. This age group is projected to continue growing in Africa, reaching an estimated 30% of the population by 2050.

Europe, on the other hand, has a relatively older population, with a median age of 42.7 years in 2020. The proportion of the population between the ages of 15 and 25 in Europe is lower than in Africa. In 2020, approximately 11% of Europe's population was between the ages of 15 and 24.

South America has a younger population compared to Europe, but not as young as Africa. The median age in South America is 32.5 years. In 2020, approximately 17% of South America's population was between the ages of 15 and 24.

Asia is the largest continent and is home to diverse countries with varying levels of economic development and demographic trends. In general, the median age in Asia is around 30 years. According to the United Nations, in 2020, approximately 15% of Asia's population was between the ages of 15 and 24.

In general, many countries and regions across the world are experiencing an aging population, which means that the proportion of older adults (typically defined as age 65 and over) is increasing relative to younger age groups. This trend is largely driven by declining fertility rates and improvements in healthcare, which have led to longer life expectancies.

Within each continent, there may be significant variation in age distribution trends depending on factors such as economic development, social policies, and cultural norms. For example, some countries in Asia, such as Japan and South Korea, are experiencing particularly rapid population aging due to low fertility rates and high life expectancies, while others, such as India and Indonesia, still have relatively young populations.

Asia has the largest population of any continent and has experienced significant changes in its age profile since 1950. In 1950, the population was young, with 46% of the population under the age of 15 and just 4% over the age of 65. However, as healthcare and living standards improved, fertility rates began to decline, leading to a shift in the age profile of the population.

By 2020, the percentage of the population under the age of 15 had declined to 25%, while that over the age of 65 had increased to 9%. The working-age population, between the ages of 15 and 64, had grown significantly, making up 66% of the population.

These changes have had significant implications for Asian societies, particularly in terms of healthcare and social welfare. As the population has aged, there has been increased demand for healthcare services and retirement support. Additionally, there has been concern about a potential labour shortage in the future, as the working-age population may not be large enough to support the needs of an aging population.

Africa has also experienced significant changes in its age profile since 1950. In 1950, the population was young, with 42% of the population under the age of 15 and just 3% over the age of 65. However, as healthcare and living standards improved, fertility rates began to decline, leading to a shift in the age profile of the population.

By 2020, the percentage of the African population under the age of 15 had declined to 38%, while the percentage of the population over the age of 65 had increased to 3%. The working-age population had also grown, making up 59% of the population.

These changes have had significant implications for African societies, particularly in terms of education and employment. As the population has grown, there has been increased demand for educational opportunities and job opportunities. Additionally, there has been concern about a potential youth bulge, as a large young population may lead to increased social unrest if job opportunities are not available.

Europe has experienced significant changes in its age profile since 1950, particularly due to a decline in fertility rates and improvements in healthcare. In 1950, the population was relatively young, with 34% of the population under the age of 15 and just 7% over the age of 65.

By 2020, the percentage of the population under the age of 15 had declined to 15%, while the percentage of the population over the age of 65 had increased to 20%. The working-age population had also declined, making up 65% of the population.

These changes have had significant implications for European societies, particularly in terms of healthcare and social welfare. As the population has aged, there has been increased demand for healthcare services and retirement support. Populist measures to lower the age of retirement and boost retirement incomes alongside increasing levels of young people delaying entry to the workforce by enrolling in further and higher education have seen the ratio of 'working-age contributors' to 'supported' citizens declining steadily with inevitable consequences for public finances.

North America too has experienced significant changes in its age profile since 1950, particularly due to improvements in healthcare and changes in fertility rates. In 1950, the population was relatively young, with 36% of the population under the age of 15 and just 6% over the age of 65. By 2020, 18% of the US population was under 15 and over 17% were over 65 years of age.

1.3 What can Influence Population Size?

Political interference in fertility rates as evidenced by family size is notoriously difficult to calculate but the enforced 'one-child' policy of China implemented between 1979 and 2015 has had a profound impact on social structures. Designed as a temporary measure to put a brake on population growth and facilitate economic growth under a planned economy, the one-child policy is responsible for 100 million one-child families, and as the support ratio declines it is clear that population aging in China is a burden not only for Chinese society but also for many of the working-age population who are the only child and may have total responsibility for two aging parents and four aged grandparents. Furthermore, three decades of the one-child policy in a society where sons were culturally more highly valued than daughters have resulted in a distorted sex ratio (Figures 1.3 and 1.4) and China now has a large pool of 20–40 million surplus young men. It is now clear that fertility rates were declining in China before the one-child policy was enforced and now, after relaxation, one child generally remains the norm as urban couples face the characteristically 'Western' problems of prolonged education, a competitive labour market, challenging career pathways, and expensive and scarce housing.

Other societies in East Asia like Japan, South Korea, Taiwan and Hong Kong have experienced similar fertility declines and have had little success in boosting their fertility even with pronatalist and pro-family policies. The essential entry of women into the (paid) labour market has obviously contributed to this situation and childlessness has become the default option for some.

India has overtaken China as the world's most populous country (1.4286 billion compared to 1.4257 billion — 2023 projections) and its population is projected to continue growing till the end of the century with 1.53 billion people whereas China's population is predicted to decline to 766 million.

This is entirely accounted for by the age distribution of the two countries. Adults aged 65 and older comprise only 7% of India's population compared to 14% in China (and 18% in the US). People under the age of 25 account for more than 40% of India's population and *globally* one in five people who are under the age of 25 live in India.

Indian women's fertility rate has been falling progressively: currently 2 children per woman compared to 3.4 in 1992 and 5.9 in 1950. There are significant differences between states, rural compared to urban, and by religion, with generally the differences accounted for by economic opportunities, health and quality of life.

India's mass sterilisation drive of 1976 which lasted during the 21-month period of the 'Emergency' resulted in over 6 million vasectomies and 2 million tubal ligations, but the backlash against effectively compulsory vasectomies was so severe that female sterilisation rapidly re-established itself as the most popular method with about 37% of women having the operation. As in China, the sex ratio is distorted by the preference for boy babies and the harsh economic consequences of having daughters, especially in rural communities (Figures 1.3 and 1.4).

In Japan, the world's third largest economy, deaths have outpaced births for more than a decade and the country also has one of the highest life expectancies in the world contributing to a ballooning elderly population. Political measures to incentivise procreation, enhance opportunities for inward migration for some foreign workers

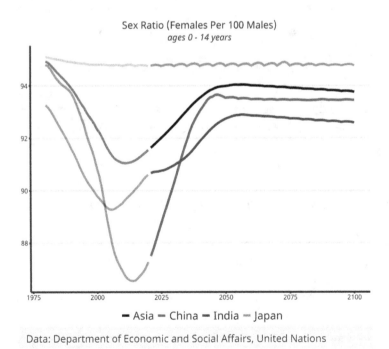

Sex Ratio (Females Per 100 Males)
ages 0 - 14 years

━ Asia ━ China ━ India ━ Japan

Data: Department of Economic and Social Affairs, United Nations

Figure 1.3   Impact of population control measures in Asia.

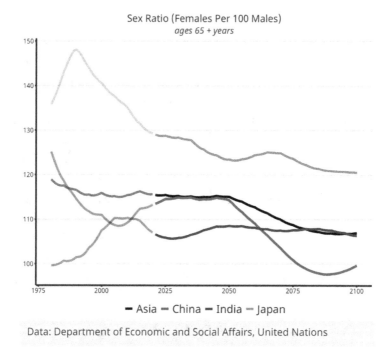

Figure 1.4 Sex ratios in aging populations.

and even the development of robots to assist with the chores of elderly care have had little impact on a society which is shrinking and aging at a concerning rate.

1.4 The Impact of Delaying and Deferring

It has been universally recognised that delaying a first pregnancy has a significant impact not only on women's health and well-being, but also on population growth and structure.

In the 1950s, in the OECD (Organisation for Economic Co-operation and Development) countries the average age of first pregnancy was around 23 years old. By the 1970s, this had increased to around 25 years old, and by the 2010s, the average age of first pregnancy was around 30 years old (Figure 1.5).

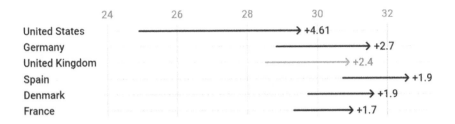

Chart: The Times and The Sunday Times • Source: Eurostat, Office of National Statistics

Figure 1.5   Age at first maternity.

This trend has been driven by several factors, including improvements in healthcare, increased access to contraception, and changes in social attitudes towards marriage and parenthood.

Europe has seen some of the highest increases in the age of first pregnancy since 1950. In the 1950s, the average age of first pregnancy in Europe was around 24 years old. By the 2010s, this had increased to around 30 years old.

This change has been driven by similar factors as in the other OECD countries, including improvements in healthcare, increased access to contraception, and changes in social attitudes towards marriage and parenthood. Additionally, the rise of feminism and the women's rights movement has played a significant role in changing attitudes towards motherhood and encouraging women to pursue their own goals before starting a family.

Asia has also seen significant increases in the age of first pregnancy since 1950, although the trend has been less pronounced than in Europe and the OECD countries. In the 1950s, the average age of first pregnancy in Asia was around 22 years old. By the 2010s, this had increased to around 26 years old.

This change has been driven by the same factors identified in Europe and the OECD countries, including improvements in healthcare, increased access to contraception, and changes in social attitudes towards marriage and parenthood. However, in some parts of Asia, traditional cultural attitudes towards motherhood and gender roles continue to play a significant role in shaping attitudes towards pregnancy and childbirth.

Africa has seen more modest increases in the age of first pregnancy since 1950, with the average age rising from around 20 years old in the 1950s to around 23 years old in the 2010s. This is largely due to lower levels of access to healthcare and education for women, as well as cultural attitudes towards motherhood and gender roles.

However, there have been some positive developments in recent years, with increased investment in healthcare and education for women, as well as campaigns to encourage family planning and improve access to contraception. These efforts have helped to raise the age of first pregnancy and improve maternal and child health outcomes in many parts of Africa.

Alongside changes in age at first pregnancy, childhood mortality and extending life expectancy, population dynamics have been influenced by the proportion of women choosing childlessness or remaining childless.

After the recognised impact of the First World War, the proportion of childless women in the UK has undergone significant changes by age since 1940. In general, there has been a gradual increase in the proportion of childless women, particularly among those in their 30s and 40s, due to factors such as increased education and career opportunities, changing attitudes towards motherhood, and improvements in contraception.

In the 1940s, the proportion of childless women in the UK was relatively low across all age groups. For example, among women aged 30–34, only around 5% were childless. However, by the 1960s and 1970s, this began to change, and the proportion of childless women increased. Among women aged 30–34 in the 1970s, around 10% were childless, and this increased to around 15% by the 1990s.

The proportion of childless women has continued to increase in the 21st century. Among women aged 30–34 in the 2000s, around 20% were childless, and this increased to around 25% by the 2010s. Among women aged 35–39, the proportion of childless women increased from around 15% in the 1990s to around 20% in the 2010s.

The proportion of childless women has also increased among those aged 40 and over. In the 1940s and 1950s, very few women in this age group were childless, but by the 2010s, around 30% of women aged 40–44 were childless. Among women aged 45–49, the proportion of childless women increased from around 10% in the 1940s to around 20% in the 2010s.

These trends can be explained by a range of factors. Firstly, women today have more opportunities for education and employment, and many choose to pursue these before starting a family. Additionally, the changing social norms have resulted in a shift towards viewing motherhood as a choice rather than an expectation. Moreover, advancements in contraception have made it easier for women to plan and control their family size.

1.5 Employment and Education have the Greatest Impact

Perhaps the most significant influence on fertility and hence family size has been women's access to the (paid) labour force. Medieval historians attest that the high death toll of the Black Death (approximately 40%) was largely responsible for incorporating women into paid agrarian labour and this resulted in delayed family initiation and smaller family sizes. Seven hundred years later, female employment patterns still dictate age at first maternity and hence family size.

Female employment rates have undergone significant changes since 1950 in countries and continents across the world driven by a range of social, economic, and cultural factors, including changes in gender roles, educational opportunities, and government policies.

In Europe, female employment rates have increased steadily since the 1950s. In 1950, the average female employment rate in Europe was just 27%, but by 2010, it had increased to over 60%. This increase was largely driven by changes in social attitudes towards women in the workplace and the expansion of education and employment opportunities for women.

In North America, female employment rates also increased significantly over the same period. In 1950, the average female employment rate in the United States was just 29%, but by 2010, it had risen to over 60%. This increase was mainly due to the growth of the service sector, changes in government policies towards women in the workplace, and the increasing numbers of women entering higher education.

In Asia, female employment rates have been more mixed. In some countries, such as Japan, female employment rates have remained relatively low, with many women opting to leave the workforce after having children. However, in other countries such as China, female employment rates have increased significantly in recent years. In 1950, the average female employment rate in China was just 17%, but by 2010, it had risen to over 65%. This increase was driven by government policies designed to encourage women to enter the workforce, as well as changes in social attitudes towards women's roles in society.

In Africa, female (paid) employment rates have been relatively low compared to other regions. In 1950, the average female employment rate in Africa was just 14%, and by 2010 it had only increased to around 30%. This slow growth can be attributed to limited education and employment opportunities for women, cultural and religious beliefs, and gender discrimination.

In Latin America, female employment rates have increased significantly since the 1950s. In 1950, the average female employment rate in Latin America was just 21%, but by 2010, it had increased to over 50%. This increase was driven by a range of factors, including changes in government policies towards women in the workforce, increasing numbers of women entering higher education, and the growth of the service sector.

In conclusion, when we ask, 'Where have all the babies gone?', the answer is overwhelmingly that women simply chose not to have them. Among the 'developed' nations, as women gained access to higher education and employment opportunities, and as social attitudes towards women's roles in society continued to evolve, motherhood came to be seen as an option and not necessarily an imperative. In the developing world, the biggest drivers for population control continue to be access for girls to education, expectations of continued reductions in childhood mortality and access to health and contraceptive care.

The biological implication is clear. Babies are not an internationally tradeable commodity. A shortage in one part of the (richer) world cannot be compensated for by an 'excess' in some other, poorer parts. Given the age profiles and current reproductive rates of the different continents, it is clear that some equilibrium may be reached by managed migration and education but political attempts thus far to deal with this 'problem' have failed and future optimism should be guarded.

Reference

All data unless otherwise cited have been obtained from United Nations sources.

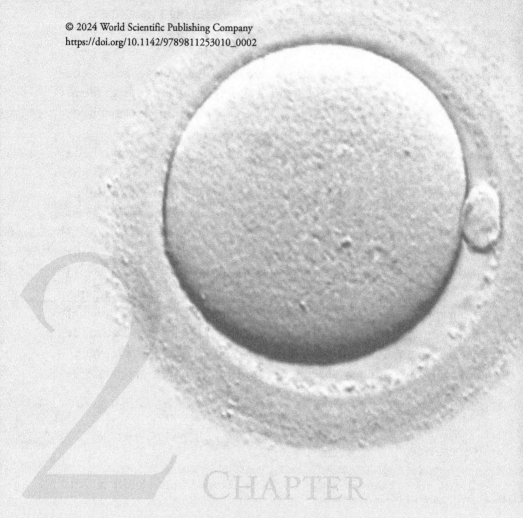

CHAPTER

History and Development
of Oocyte Cryopreservation

Georgios Petsas

2.1 Introduction

When one considers the history of gamete cryobiology, it is difficult to select a specific point of origin. Almost 360 years ago, Robert Boyle published a monograph titled *New Experiments and Observations Touching Cold* or *An Experimental History of Cold* (Leibo, 2004). Although the objective of prolonged storage of tissues that could be revitalised following suspended animation in cryostorage was envisioned over three centuries ago, oocyte cryopreservation has only quite recently become an important component of human-assisted reproductive technology.

2.2 A Brief History of Mammalian Gamete/Embryo Cryobiology

Numerous references place the beginning of cryobiology in 1776, when the Italian physiologist Spallanzani documented the observation that human spermatozoa became immotile when cooled in snow. Less than 100 years later another Italian scientist, Montegazza, proposed a sperm bank as a practical means of transporting frozen bovine spermatozoa. He even suggested that the method might be applicable to the storing of human sperm, in which case soldiers away at war would be able to have progeny (Leibo, 2004). Despite the numerous empirical studies on mammalian spermatozoa cryopreservation in the 1930s and 1940s, a major breakthrough in cryobiology occurred in 1949 with Polge's accidental discovery of the cryoprotective properties of glycerol for human spermatozoa (Polge et al, 1949). In the early 1950s, investigations on cryopreservation of rabbit oocytes and embryos (Chang, 1952) paved the way for studies on cryopreservation of female gametes and embryos. In the following years, the use of glycerol had also been explored in attempts to cryopreserve mouse (Sherman & Lin, 1959) and sheep (Averill & Rowson, 1959) unfertilised oocytes and rabbit-fertilised oocytes (Smith, 1953) with little success. It was in the 1960s when basic study investigations on cell-specific optimal freezing and warming rates set the foundation for future cryobiology (Mazur, 1970). Then in the 1970s, Whittingham et al (1972) reported the successful cryopreservation of mouse embryos using dimethyl sulfoxide (DMSO) as a cryoprotective agent (CPA) combined with a slow freezing rate and storage in liquid nitrogen. The potential benefits of cryopreservation of mature oocytes over embryos prompted the application of the procedure previously developed for freezing of mouse embryos to freezing of mouse mature oocytes (Whittingham, 1977). Following the live birth of offspring from cryopreserved mouse oocytes in 1977 (Whittingham, 1977), application of the same methodologies of cryopreservation in the early 1980s led to the establishment of the first human pregnancies after embryo cryopreservation at the cleavage stage (Trounson & Mohr, 1983). Finally, Chen (1986) reported the first pregnancy after human oocyte cryopreservation. It is of interest that slow freezing protocols established in these studies continue to be used for oocyte cryopreservation even today.

2.3 History of Human Oocyte Cryopreservation

In contrast to embryo freezing, oocyte cryopreservation has been largely neglected until quite recently. Legislative restrictions and ethical concerns regarding the production and freezing of supernumerary embryos somewhat accelerated the research into oocyte cryopreservation, leading to significant technical advances (milestones summarised in Table 2.1).

Successful pregnancies from frozen oocytes were first achieved in the late 1980s, using slow-freeze and rapid-thaw cryopreservation techniques (Chen, 1986; van Uem et al, 1987; Al-Hasani et al, 1987). In 1986, Chen reported the first pregnancy resulting in the live birth of twins using DMSO and, a year later, Van Uem et al and Al-Hasani et al reported a live birth and two pregnancies which resulted in

Table 2.1   Milestones in cryopreservation of human oocytes.

	Year	Author(s)
1st birth from DMSO-based slow freezing	1986	Chen
1st birth from PROH-based slow freezing	1997	Porcu et al
1st pregnancy from vitrified oocytes	1999	Cha et al
1st birth from vitrified oocytes	1999	Kuleshova et al
1st birth from 'Cryotop' vitrification	2005	Kyono et al

abortion, respectively. Although in Chen's hands the DMSO-based freezing resulted in good survival, fertilisation and cleavage rates (80%, 83% and 60%, respectively), other groups not only failed to achieve equally good results after freezing and thawing of human oocytes but also reported a polyploidy rate up to 40% (Al-Hasani et al, 1987; Mandelbaum et al, 1988).

Even more inconsistent were the results of studies comparing slow freezing with 1,2-propanediol (PROH) as a CPA and DMSO-based vitrification (Al-Hasani et al, 1987; Mandelbaum et al, 1988; Pensis et al, 1989; Trounson, 1986) with the latter reporting a survival rate ranging from 4% to 60%. These inconsistent results, together with concerns regarding normality following oocyte cryopreservation, brought clinical oocyte cryopreservation to a halt.

In the 1990s, despite improvement in survival rates with the DMSO procedure, human oocytes failed to progress past fertilisation (Hunter et al, 1991). The good survival and blastulation rate for mouse pronuclear zygotes with the modified method to include 0.1 M sucrose PROH, and the similarity in the estimated water permeability for the mouse pronuclear zygote and the human metaphase-II oocyte, led to this method being assessed for human oocytes. The immediate post-thaw survival rate observed was over 60% (Gook et al, 1993). Equally promising was the developmental potential of these oocytes. The observations of a protective action of PROH on the spindle and of an abundance of cortical granules within the oocyte suggested that the fertilisation potential was unimpaired (Gook et al, 1993).

Confirming this suggestion, a similar normal fertilisation rate to that for non-frozen oocytes inseminated with the same sperm preparation was observed for the cryopreserved oocytes with no increase in haploidy or polyploidy (Gook et al, 1994). The next challenge, to determine whether normal embryo development was possible, was alleviated in 1995 by the confirmation of embryo development to the blastocyst stage following intracytoplasmic sperm injection (Gook et al, 1995) and the establishment in 1996 of three pregnancies using PROH (Tucker et al, 1996). Despite none of these pregnancies continuing to term, normal karyotype was indicated (Tucker et al, 1996). In February 1997, the Bologna group reported the first birth following oocyte freeze with PROH and intracytoplasmic sperm injection (Porcu et al, 1997). Although not included in the original goals, the application of intracytoplasmic sperm injection as an elective technique for cryopreserved oocytes was found to rectify fertilisation issues due to zona pellucida hardening and has opened the gate for widespread application of oocyte cryopreservation.

2.4 Evolution of Methods for Oocyte Cryopreservation

Oocyte cryopreservation has evolved significantly since the first achieved human pregnancy. There are two basic techniques applied to the cryopreservation of human oocytes: controlled slow freezing, which was favoured in early protocols, and ultrarapid cooling by vitrification, which is now well established. Slow freezing results in a liquid changing to a solid state whereas vitrification results in a non-crystalline amorphous solid.

2.4.1 Slow Freezing

During slow freezing, cells are exposed to a low concentration of CPAs and slow decreases in temperature. Oocytes are first cooled to a temperature of –5°C to –7°C, at which equilibration and seeding take place. Oocytes are then cooled at a slow rate of 0.3–0.5°C/minute, until a temperature of between –30°C and –65°C has been reached, before being added to liquid nitrogen for storage. Since its introduction and first success obtained in the 1980s using DMSO as a CPA, this cryopreservation method has been extensively revisited and modified to improve laboratory and clinical results. In an attempt to enhance the level of dehydration, increasing the sucrose concentration to 0.2 or 0.3 M was suggested. Fabbri et al (2001) found that doubling the sucrose concentration to 0.2 M resulted in a statistically significant increase in oocyte survival (60% vs 34%), which was even higher (82%) if the concentration was tripled to 0.3 M. The scientific community welcomed these encouraging results and many groups soon adopted the high sucrose concentration protocol. From a number of studies published in 2006–2007, it appeared that using 0.2 M compared to 0.1 M sucrose resulted in better statistics (survival rate: 72% vs 50%; fertilisation rate: 80% vs 54%; cleavage rate: 93% vs 85%, respectively). Similarly, clinical outcomes were better in the 0.2 M than in the 0.1 M sucrose group (implantation rate: 17% vs 10%) (Gook & Edgar, 2007). Despite improvements in the laboratory outcomes, it appeared that the implantation potential of the resultant embryos in the 0.3 M sucrose group was compromised due to perturbations of the cytoplasm and degeneration of mitochondria.

In a similar attempt to increase the oocyte survival rate while supporting its developmental competence, removal of sodium from the cryopreservation media and substitution with choline was introduced (Quintans et al, 2002). Despite the hypothesis that choline may act as a stabiliser of cell membranes furnishing protection against freezing damage, data obtained from choline-based freezing media did not suggest improved outcomes compared with more conventional media (Edgar & Gook, 2012).

Although survival of slow-frozen oocytes was improved over the years through a fine restatement of the original freezing protocol, concerns surrounding the clinical efficiency of this technique

(Edgar & Gook, 2012) resulted in shifting from slow freezing to an alternative strategy.

2.4.2 Vitrification

Even though the possibility of vitrified water was proposed by Brayley (1860), the earliest suggestion that vitrification might be an appropriate strategy for cryopreservation came from Stiles (1930). Luyet (1937) is widely acknowledged as being the first to take to heart the idea of vitrification of living cells but it took almost 50 years for Rall and Fahy (1985) to be able to close the gap between theory and practice, and confirm the universality of the fundamental principles of vitrification by successfully applying lessons learned from adult rabbit kidneys to the vitrification of eight-cell mouse embryos.

In essence, vitrification involves equilibration of the specimen in a cocktail of CPAs followed by plunging into liquid nitrogen. It normally requires molar concentrations threefold or fourfold higher than for slow freezing, and a very rapid rate of cooling below the glass transition temperature. Rewarming must also be ultrarapid to avoid ice nucleation. The major drawbacks of the technology are toxicity from the high solute concentrations — biochemical and osmotic — for which there are various strategies for mitigation. Ishimori et al (1993) suggested that reducing the duration of exposure to vitrification solutions reduced the toxicity. This appeared to improve survival of human vitrified oocytes but embryonic cell division and further development were inhibited (Hunter et al, 1995). As had been the case with slow freezing, this prompted a transition from DMSO-based vitrification solutions in favour of ethylene glycol (EG). The EG-based solution developed by Ali and Shelton (1993) was proved successful for bovine (Martino et al, 1996) and murine (Hotamisligil et al, 1996) oocytes and resulted in the first pregnancy (Cha, 1999) and birth (Kuleshova et al, 1999) from vitrified oocytes. Based on Rall and Fahy's original philosophy of using a combination of CPAs to reduce individual toxicities, the combination of EG and DMSO became, by the end of the 1990s, the basis of the vitrification revolution in assisted reproduction treatment resulting in pregnancies from vitrified blastocysts (Vanderzwalmen et al, 1997) and births from vitrified cleavage-stage embryos (Hsieh et al, 1999). For human oocytes, however, both the use of a single cryoprotectant (EG) and a combination of cryoprotectants (EG+DMSO) together with sucrose continued to be used for many years, causing cryobiologists who have laboured over the science for years to lament: 'After years of experience, the choice of compositions utilised still seems nearly random, and little consensus seems to exist as to which solutions are optimal for which reproductive cells' (Mullen & Fahy, 2011).

There was, however, no disagreement about the importance of cooling at the fastest possible rate to guarantee vitrification and avoid cryodamage. Because cooling rates vary inversely with the mass of the specimen, a number of devices have been invented for vitrifying oocytes. After the first experience with traditional straws (0.25 mL), which revealed their unsuitableness, it was suggested to use new devices guaranteeing minimal volume loading (1 µL). Since then, a number of different cryo-tools have been proposed, till the introduction by Kuwayama et al (2005) of the widely used 'Cryotop' technique. By achieving an extremely rapid cooling rate, facilitated by minimal fluid volume, survival rates of over 90% and the establishment of live births were reported (Kyono et al, 2005). Due to its technically challenging nature, the Cryotop was originally slow to gain widespread acceptance for oocyte vitrification but minor methodological modifications and a large comparative study (Cobo et al, 2008) cemented its place in oocyte cryopreservation history (Gobo, 2011). This and many other so-called "open systems" that assure extremely rapid direct contact with liquid nitrogen have been successfully used, including modified straws, capillaries, and nylon loops. Despite their proven proficiency, concerns have been raised over the sterility of open systems due to potential cross-contamination between the vitrification sample and liquid nitrogen. The demand from regulatory authorities like the U.S. Food and Drug Administration for greater safety has led to the introduction of "closed systems" that supply a physical barrier between the sample and liquid nitrogen, providing theoretically heightened biosafety. However, the use of closed systems raised new concerns about the efficiency of oocyte vitrification, due to their decreased cooling rates that can potentially hamper the final laboratory and clinical outcomes (Vajta et al, 2015). Till today, the choice to use closed rather than open systems is strongly debated.

2.4.3 The Trend Towards Vitrification

Since the first reported success with human vitrified oocytes (Kuleshova et al, 1999), several studies have stated the superiority of vitrification over slow freezing and its noninferiority compared with fresh cycles. In a meta-analysis, Cobo & Diaz (2011) reported that the rates of survival, fertilisation, embryo cleavage, top-quality embryos and ongoing pregnancy were higher in the vitrification group and also that fertilisation, embryo cleavage, and ongoing pregnancy rates did not differ between vitrification and fresh oocyte groups. This led to a widespread shift to vitrification by many groups as a technique to cryopreserve oocytes and a 2013 update to the National Institute for Health and Care Excellence guidelines that state: 'In cryopreservation of oocytes and embryos, use vitrification instead of controlled-rate freezing if the necessary equipment and expertise is available' (National Collaborating Centre for Women's and Children's Health (UK), 2013). Whereas in 1999, close to 100 cryopreserved oocytes were needed to achieve one pregnancy (Porcu, 1999), in 2015 the largest reported series to date of women undergoing elective oocyte cryopreservation for non-oncologic reasons showed that the optimal number of stored vitrified oocytes to achieve a pregnancy was only 8–10 and that pregnancy rates were age-dependent (Cobo et al, 2016).

2.5 Oocyte Cryopreservation: From Research to Regulatory Guidelines

Although it has taken many years since the first birth from a frozen oocyte was achieved, the acceptance of oocyte cryopreservation in general assisted reproduction practice has finally come to fruition, having answered many of the criticisms raised during a chequered past. Soon after the first birth from vitrified oocytes, in 2000, the Human Fertilisation and Embryology Authority (HFEA) allowed the use of frozen oocytes for infertility treatment in the UK (Wise, 2000). In 2002, the UK welcomed the first birth from frozen oocytes but only almost 20 years later, the HFEA increased the statutory storage limit for frozen gametes and embryos from 10 years to a 10-year renewable period up to a maximum of 55 years.

Whilst oocyte cryopreservation was initially reserved for women with medical indications who had no other fertility options (ESHRE Task Force on Ethics and Law, 2004), in 2012 the European Society for Human Reproduction and Embryology (ESHRE) considered oocyte cryopreservation also acceptable for age-related fertility decline (ESHRE Task Force on Ethics and Law, 2012), resulting in 'social egg freezing' becoming a popular subject within the media with a growing debate surrounding its use.

Finally, in 2013, following increasing evidence about the noninferiority of *in vitro* fertilisation using vitrified oocytes compared to *in vitro* fertilisation with fresh oocytes, the American Society for Reproductive Medicine lifted the experimental label from modern procedures to cryopreserve oocytes, stating, however, that 'there are not yet sufficient data to recommend oocyte cryopreservation for the sole purpose of circumventing reproductive aging in healthy women' (Practice Committees of the American Society for Reproductive Medicine and the Society for Assisted Reproductive Technology, 2013).

2.6 Future of Oocyte Cryobiology

When one thinks back in history, it is remarkable to consider that the advancements in cryopreservation of gametes are based, at least philosophically, on techniques pioneered by the likes of Polge in the 1950s. So, what might one expect in the future? It is a fool's errand to make sweeping predictions because a breakthrough often comes unexpectedly, as it did for Polge over 70 years ago. Nevertheless, it seems safe to forecast that advances in two fields, genomics and information science, may provide currently inconceivable advancements that, once applied, will transform the future for fertility preservation. Cutting-edge techniques to unveil the molecular alterations — epigenetic, proteomic and transcriptomic — exerted by cryopreservation and hybrid artificial intelligence models allowing accurate quantification of the oocyte developmental competence will hopefully help pregnancy and live birth rates climb asymptotically in the future.

References

Al-Hasani S, Diedrich K, van der Ven H, Reinecke A, Hartje M, Krebs D. Cryopreservation of human oocytes. Hum Reprod. 1987 Nov;2(8): 695–700.

Ali J, Shelton JN. Design of vitrification solutions for the cryopreservation of embryos. J Reprod Fertil. 1993 Nov;99(2):471–7.

Averill RLW, Rowson LEA. Attempts at storage of sheep ova at low temperatures. J Agric Sci. 1959;52(3):392–5.

Brayley EW. II. Notes on the apparent universality of a principle analogous to regelation, on the physical nature of glass, and on the probable existence of water in a state corresponding to that of glass. Proc R Soc Lond. 1860;10:450–60.

Cha KY. Pregnancy and implantation from vitrified oocytes following in vitro fertilization (IVF) and in vitro culture (IVC). Fertil Steril. 1999; 72(1):S2.

Chang MC. Fertilizability of rabbit ova and the effects of temperature in vitro on their subsequent fertilization and activation in vivo. J Exp Zool. 1952;121:351–81.

Chen C. Pregnancy after human oocyte cryopreservation. Lancet. 1986 Apr 19;1(8486):884–6.

Cobo A, Diaz C. Clinical application of oocyte vitrification: a systematic review and meta-analysis of randomized controlled trials. Fertil Steril. 2011 Aug;96(2):277–85.

Cobo A, García-Velasco JA, Coello A, Domingo J, Pellicer A, Remohí J. Oocyte vitrification as an efficient option for elective fertility preservation. Fertil Steril. 2016 Mar;105(3):755–764.e8.

Cobo A, Kuwayama M, Pérez S, Ruiz A, Pellicer A, Remohí J. Comparison of concomitant outcome achieved with fresh and cryopreserved donor oocytes vitrified by the Cryotop method. Fertil Steril. 2008 Jun;89(6):1657–64.

Edgar DH, Gook DA. A critical appraisal of cryopreservation (slow cooling versus vitrification) of human oocytes and embryos. Hum Reprod Update. 2012 Sep-Oct;18(5):536–54.

ESHRE Task Force on Ethics and Law. Taskforce 7: Ethical considerations for the cryopreservation of gametes and reproductive tissues for self use. Hum Reprod. 2004 Feb;19(2):460–2.

ESHRE Task Force on Ethics and Law; Dondorp W, de Wert G, Pennings G, Shenfield F, Devroey P, Tarlatzis B, Barri P, Diedrich K. Oocyte cryopreservation for age-related fertility loss. Hum Reprod. 2012 May;27(5):1231–7.

Fabbri R, Porcu E, Marsella T, Rocchetta G, Venturoli S, Flamigni C. Human oocyte cryopreservation: new perspectives regarding oocyte survival. Hum Reprod. 2001 Mar;16(3):411–6.

Gook DA, Edgar DH. Human oocyte cryopreservation. Hum Reprod Update. 2007 Nov-Dec;13(6):591–605.

Gook DA, Osborn SM, Bourne H, Johnston WI. Fertilization of human oocytes following cryopreservation; normal karyotypes and absence of stray chromosomes. Hum Reprod. 1994 Apr;9(4):684–91.

Gook DA, Osborn SM, Johnston WI. Cryopreservation of mouse and human oocytes using 1,2-propanediol and the configuration of the meiotic spindle. Hum Reprod. 1993 Jul;8(7):1101–9.

Gook DA, Schiewe MC, Osborn SM, Asch RH, Jansen RP, Johnston WI. Intracytoplasmic sperm injection and embryo development of human oocytes cryopreserved using 1,2-propanediol. Hum Reprod. 1995 Oct;10(10):2637–41.

Gook DA. History of oocyte cryopreservation. Reprod Biomed Online. 2011 Sep;23(3):281–9.

Hotamisligil S, Toner M, Powers RD. Changes in membrane integrity, cytoskeletal structure, and developmental potential of murine oocytes after vitrification in ethylene glycol. Biol Reprod. 1996 Jul;55(1):161–8.

Hsieh YY, Tsai HD, Chang CC, Chang CC, Lo HY, Lai AC. Ultrarapid cryopreservation of human embryos: experience with 1,582 embryos. Fertil Steril. 1999 Aug;72(2):253–6.

Hunter JE, Bernard A, Fuller B, Amso N, Shaw RW. Fertilization and development of the human oocyte following exposure to cryoprotectants, low temperatures and cryopreservation: a comparison of two techniques. Hum Reprod. 1991 Nov;6(10):1460–5.

Hunter JE, Fuller BJ, Bernard A, Jackson A, Shaw RW. Vitrification of human oocytes following minimal exposure to cryoprotectants; initial studies on fertilization and embryonic development. Hum Reprod. 1995 May;10(5):1184–8.

Ishimori H, Saeki K, Inai M, Nagao Y, Itasaka J, Miki Y, Seike N, Kainuma H. Vitrification of bovine embryos in a mixture of ethylene glycol and dimethyl sulfoxide. Theriogenology. 1993 Aug;40(2):427–33.

Kuleshova L, Gianaroli L, Magli C, Ferraretti A, Trounson A. Birth following vitrification of a small number of human oocytes: case report. Hum Reprod. 1999 Dec;14(12):3077–9.

Kuwayama M, Vajta G, Kato O, Leibo SP. Highly efficient vitrification method for cryopreservation of human oocytes. Reprod Biomed Online. 2005 Sep;11(3):300–8.

Kyono K, Fuchinoue K, Yagi A, Nakajo Y, Yamashita A, Kumagai S. Successful pregnancy and delivery after transfer of a single blastocyst derived from a vitrified mature human oocyte. Fertil Steril. 2005 Oct;84(4):1017.

Leibo SP. The early history of gamete cryobiology. In: Fuller BJ, Lane N, Benson EE, editors. Life in the frozen state. CRC Press; 2004. p. 373–96.

Luyet, BJ. The vitrification of organic colloids and of protoplasme. Biodynamica. 1937;1(29):1–14.

Mandelbaum J, Junca AM, Plachot M, Alnot MO, Salat-Baroux J, Alvarez S, Tibi C, Cohen J, Debache C, Tesquier L. Cryopreservation of human embryos and oocytes. Hum Reprod. 1988 Jan;3(1):117–9.

Martino A, Songsasen N, Leibo SP. Development into blastocysts of bovine oocytes cryopreserved by ultra-rapid cooling. Biol Reprod. 1996 May;54(5):1059–69.

Mazur P. Cryobiology: the freezing of biological systems. Science. 1970 May 22;168(3934):939–49.

Mullen SF, Fahy GM. Fundamental aspects of vitrification as a method of reproductive cell, tissue and organ cryopreservation. In: Donnez J, Kim SS, editors. Principles and practice of fertility preservation. Cambridge University Press; 2011. p. 145–163.

National Collaborating Centre for Women's and Children's Health (UK). Fertility: Assessment and Treatment for People with Fertility Problems. London: Royal College of Obstetricians & Gynaecologists; 2013 Feb. PMID: 25340218.

Pensis M, Loumaye E, Psalti I. Screening of conditions for rapid freezing of human oocytes: preliminary study toward their cryopreservation. Fertil Steril. 1989 Nov;52(5):787–94.

Polge C, Smith AU, Parkes AS. Revival of spermatozoa after vitrification and dehydration at low temperatures. Nature. 1949 Oct 15;164(4172):666.

Porcu E, Fabbri R, Seracchioli R, Ciotti PM, Magrini O, Flamigni C. Birth of a healthy female after intracytoplasmic sperm injection of cryopreserved human oocytes. Fertil Steril. 1997 Oct;68(4):724–6.

Porcu E. Cycles of human oocyte cryopreservation and intracytoplasmic sperm injection: results of 112 cycles. Fertil Steril. 1999;72(Suppl. 1):S2.

Practice Committees of the American Society for Reproductive Medicine and the Society for Assisted Reproductive Technology. Mature oocyte cryopreservation: a guideline. Fertil Steril. 2013 Jan;99(1):37–43.

Quintans CJ, Donaldson MJ, Bertolino MV, Pasqualini RS. Birth of two babies using oocytes that were cryopreserved in a choline-based freezing medium. Hum Reprod. 2002 Dec;17(12):3149–52.

Rall WF, Fahy GM. Ice-free cryopreservation of mouse embryos at -196 degrees C by vitrification. Nature. 1985 Feb 14–20;313(6003):573–5.

Sherman JK, Lin TP. Temperature shock and cold-storage of unfertilized mouse eggs. Fertil Steril. 1959 Jul-Aug;10(4):384–96.

Smith, AU. In vitro experiments with rabbit eggs. In: Churchill J, editor. Mammalian germ cells. Ciba Foundation Symposium; 1953. p. 217–32.

Stiles, W. On the cause of cold death of plants. Protoplasma. 1930;9(1): 459–68.

Trounson A, Mohr L. Human pregnancy following cryopreservation, thawing and transfer of an eight-cell embryo. Nature. 1983 Oct 20–26;305(5936):707–9.

Trounson A. Preservation of human eggs and embryos. Fertil Steril. 1986 Jul;46(1):1–12.

Tucker M, Wright G, Morton P, Shanguo L, Massey J, Kort H. Preliminary experience with human oocyte cryopreservation using 1,2-propanediol and sucrose. Hum Reprod. 1996 Jul;11(7):1513–5.

Vajta G, Rienzi L, Ubaldi FM. Open versus closed systems for vitrification of human oocytes and embryos. Reprod Biomed Online. 2015 Apr; 30(4):325–33.

van Uem JF, Siebzehnrübl ER, Schuh B, Koch R, Trotnow S, Lang N. Birth after cryopreservation of unfertilized oocytes. Lancet. 1987 Mar 28;1(8535):752–3.

Vanderzwalmen P, Delval A, Chatziparasidou A, Bertin G, Ectors F, Lejeune B, Nijs M, Prapas N, Prapas Y, Van Damme B, Zech H, Schoysman R. O-198. Pregnancies after vitrification of human day 5 embryos. Hum Reprod. 1997 Jun 1;12(Suppl 2):98.

Whittingham DG, Leibo SP, Mazur P. Survival of mouse embryos frozen to -196 degrees and -269 degrees C. Science. 1972;178(4059):411–4.

Whittingham DG. Fertilization in vitro and development to term of unfertilized mouse oocytes previously stored at –196 degrees C. J Reprod Fertil. 1977 Jan;49(1):89–94.

Wise J. UK lifts ban on frozen eggs. BMJ. 2000 Feb 5;320(7231):334.

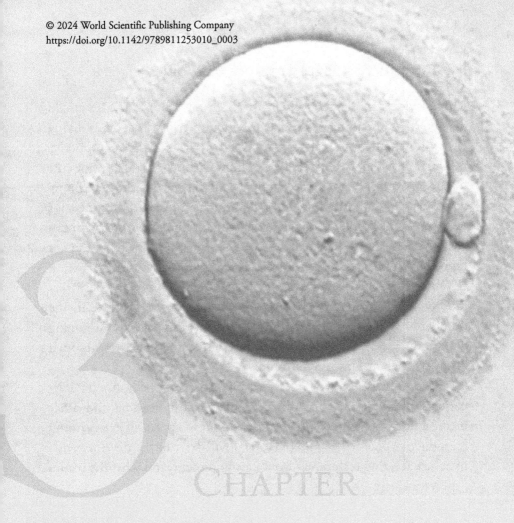

CHAPTER

Human Oocyte Freezing Technologies: Current State-of-Art and Future Perspectives

Evrim Ünsal

3.1 Introduction: The Treasure of Women

The oocyte is the largest cell in the body by volume (~110 μm in diameter). Containing all the components that will form a living structure when combined with the sperm cell, it is the reproductive treasure of women and therefore humanity. In parallel with the increasing role of women in technology and business in the developing world, having children remains a desire that must be postponed for many women. Problems can arise if a woman finds a partner who can adapt to her future life plans, but the woman's desire to become a mother may be pushed into the background as a secret passion (Donnez et al, 2021). However, the biggest limitation on her desire for motherhood is not social but biological, due to the decrease in the number of viable eggs in the ovaries with increasing age and the aging of those oocytes. This aging also increases the likelihood of chromosomal disorders such as Down Syndrome.

Oocyte freezing, which started by being applied in oncology patients and whose use has increased for social indications and other medical reasons, has become a more widespread approach in extending reproductive potential. In this chapter, I will describe the developments in oocyte freezing techniques from past to present, and what the future expectations are.

3.2 The Egg Freezing Revolution

Cryopreservation refers to the freezing of cells and tissues and the preservation of their vitality and physiological properties for future use by stopping their biological activities through storing them at sub-zero temperatures. Irreversible damage can occur when the high amounts of water in the cells turn into ice crystals.

Egg cells, which are the largest cells in the human body, are the cells most affected by the freezing process among the reproductive cells. Cells are treated with cryoprotectants so that they are not damaged during freezing, thus their viability is preserved and they can be stored for a long time. In this context, researchers have worked for years to find the most effective cryoprotectant, as well as reduce its toxic effects depending on the concentration and exposure time during application. However, while sperm and embryo freezing have become a fundamental part of *in vitro* fertilisation (IVF) applications, oocyte freezing technology — first reported in the 1980s — has not become widespread until recently, since the desired viability rates could not be achieved. Considering the indications of the patient groups included in the oocyte freezing program, it is obvious that it will not be easy to take responsibility for the reproduction possibility of cancer patients especially and cases with low ovarian reserve. Due to the high success rates achieved with the development of the vitrification technique, these problems have been largely overcome and a new glimmer of hope has appeared on the horizon for many women who want to preserve their fertility and have the chance of becoming a mother.

The first pregnancy with frozen oocytes was reported in 1986 in Australia by Chen et al. Since oocytes are very difficult cell types for cryopreservation, effective success was not achieved for many years. In addition to physiological parameters, the difficulties in determining membrane permeability, chromosomal segregation errors that may occur as a result of damage at the organelle level, and decreased fertilisation rates due to the thickening of the zona pellucida have left oocyte cryopreservation in the background among IVF applications for many years.

Cryoprotectants (CPAs), which are used to prevent cell damage due to ice crystallisation at ultra-low temperatures, play a very important role in the success of the technique. They reduce the freezing temperature, preventing cell damage not only during freezing but also during thawing. They are divided into two groups as permeating (P-CPA) and non-permeating (NP-CPA) (Table 3.1).

CPAs, which increase the elasticity of the cell membrane by affecting the lipid content, firstly cause the cell to shrink and lose

Table 3.1   Commonly used cryoprotectants.

Permeating Cryoprotectants	Non-Permeating Cryoprotectants	
	Sugars	Polymers
Dimethyl sulfoxide (DMSO)	Sucrose	Polyethylene glycol
Ethylene glycol	Trehalose	Polyvinyl pyrrolidone
Propylene glycol	Raffinose	Hydroxy ethyl starch
Glycerol	Mannitol	Ficoll
Methanol	Glucose	Serum proteins (mixture)
Ethanol	Galactose	Milk proteins (mixture)

intracellular fluid. While the CPAs diffuse into the cell, the cell fluid re-enters the cell and the cells recover their original configuration by providing the osmotic balance. It is very important to establish the balance quickly, and at this point the developmental stage of the cell is effective, as well as the high concentration and ambient temperature that increase the rate of diffusion of the cryoprotectant material through the cell membrane.

3.3 At What Developmental Stage Should the Oocyte be Frozen?

The success of cryopreservation at different meiotic stages of the oocyte also varies. Although metaphase II (MII) oocytes are commonly frozen, the focus has been on freezing germinal vesicle (GV) stage oocytes, considering spindle damage and possible aneuploidy. The fact that the nuclear material is surrounded by a membrane suggests that oocytes at the GV stage are the most suitable cell type for freezing, but low viability has led to the preference of MII oocytes in routine practice. Although these cells are at the most suitable stage for freezing due to the completion of meiosis, spindle damage is a parameter that can affect meiosis II.

3.4 What are the Challenges in Oocyte Freezing?

Low surface area/large volume ratio is one of the most important factors underlying the difficulty of oocyte freezing compared to other cell types. While the surface area/volume ratio of the sperm cell is 4.3, this ratio for oocytes is only 0.05 because they are spherical. Therefore, it needs more time to reach osmotic equilibrium and the optimum freezing point is quite low compared to other cell types. During the equilibration of CPAs, osmotic exchange between intracellular and extracellular fluids causes large changes in cell volume, which may result in cell rupture. In order to prevent this condition resulting in cell death, CPAs must be added slowly and precisely.

Although there are approaches to increase freezing success by targeting different developmental stages of the oocyte (MII or GV), cells in the MII stage are usually frozen in routine applications. The first polar body has been extruded and chromosome condensation has taken place in the oocyte at this stage, where nuclear and cytoplasmic maturation have been completed. Events that disrupt oocyte physiology can also cause oocyte damage during freezing, while the most common problem is oocyte degeneration due to oolemma breakage caused by intracellular ice formation and osmotic stress. During freezing and thawing, the wall surrounding the oocyte (zona pellucida) may thicken, and the meiotic spindle apparatus and intracellular organelles may be damaged. Additional risks include *in vitro* aging, parthenogenesis and epigenetic risks.

When the sperm comes into contact with the oolemma (oocyte membrane), intracellular Ca^{2+} increases and cortical granules become active. From these granules, lysosomal enzymes are released into the perivitelline space between the zona pellucida and oolemma, thus thickening the zona pellucida. With the membrane depolarisation that occurs, the zona pellucida thickens and does not allow the penetration of other sperm cells. Oocyte freezing causes the release of cortical granules and non-physiological zona thickening occurs. This situation, which reduces the fertilisation potential of the oocyte, supports the view that fertilisation will be more effective with intracytoplasmic sperm injection method instead of conventional IVF application in frozen oocytes. Meiotic spindles, which are sensitive to temperature differences, can be damaged during freezing and thawing. This causes aneuploidies (numerical chromosomal anomalies) to occur, since the sequencing and error-free segregation of chromosomes can only occur in the presence of meiotic spindles.

The most important dysmorphism in cryopreserved oocytes due to cryo-damage and/or osmotic stress is vacuolisation, which may present with low fertilisation rates. Organelle damage, especially of smooth endoplasmic reticulum and mitochondria, can also be seen. Apart from the cytogenetic effects of freezing, it is thought that the risk of parthenogenetic activation in oocytes may increase after CPA exposure, but current data suggest that this rate is not higher than the rate seen in fresh oocytes. The long-term effects of epigenetic changes on human health are unknown, as research on whether cryodamage in frozen oocytes can cause epigenetic changes in the embryo is still limited in animal models.

3.5 Who is Oocyte Freezing Applicable to?

The increase in the success of oocyte cryopreservation and the achievement of similar pregnancy rates with fresh embryo transfer in IVF cycles have enabled this technique to be applied to a wider indication group. Although this method was initially applied to women with medical indications who did not have any other fertility options, social egg freezing has become more widespread because of the markedly reduced chances of fertility treatment success in older women.

While oocyte freezing for donation purposes was initially applied to women who would develop only a small number of oocytes due to premature ovarian failure, it has now become widespread as a treatment preferred especially by older women. Through the use of frozen oocytes from young donors and the developments in freezing techniques, obtaining competent embryos with high viability rates and pregnancy success has enhanced convenience in ensuring the synchronisation of the donor and recipient endometrium. With the formation of donor oocyte cryobanks, the cost per cycle has decreased and the patients' ability to access treatment has increased. Cancer cases are perhaps the most important group in need of high success rates among oocyte freezing programs. When these patients learn that they have cancer, their desire to protect their future reproductive potential can be very strong and there is the need to coordinate the oncological treatment plan. In this group of patients, who often do not have time to obtain enough oocytes to perform more than one IVF attempt, it is vital to obtain a success rate of oocyte freezing and thawing close to 100%, and the goal of obtaining good-quality embryos is also a challenge for reproductive medicine professionals. Preservation of the reproductive ability of the cancer patient after oncology treatment has an important role in improving the quality of life (Table 3.2).

Apart from cancer cases, endometriosis cases with decreased ovarian reserve after surgery, women exposed to gonadotoxic treatment

Table 3.2   Oocyte cryopreservation indications.

Indications For Oocyte Cryopreservation

1. Conservation of fertility
    a. Cancer treatments that cause high-dose radiation of the pelvis
    b. Ovarian surgeries that result in infertility
    c. Male medical therapies (anti-retroviral) risking failure to obtain sperm for IVF or intracytoplasmic sperm injection on the day of oocyte retrieval
    d. Medical or surgical procedures that lead to ovarian reserve compromise
    e. Premature ovarian failure that results in reduced fertility
2. Establishment of donor oocyte banks
3. Sperm unavailability for the collection day
4. Limitations and regulations about embryo freezing
5. Social egg freezing

due to autoimmune diseases, and women with the risk of early menopause or with genetic aberrations that cause sub-fertility are among the patient groups included in oocyte freezing programs. These genetic conditions include Fragile X premutation causing primary ovarian failure and mosaic monosomies on the X chromosome. Oocyte cryopreservation, which is also used for the cryopreservation of "spare" gametes in the IVF process, is also an important application to protect the woman's eggs in the event that sperm cannot be found on the day of oocyte retrieval. If sperm is obtained from the partner with advanced treatment options, these frozen egg cells will give the woman a chance to conceive without a new induction.

3.6 Oocyte Cryopreservation Techniques

In a joint document published in 2013 by the American Society for Reproductive Medicine and the Society for Assisted Reproductive Technology, it was stated that modern techniques used in mature oocyte cryopreservation (MII) are no longer experimental and can be used in routine IVF practice (Donnez and Dolmann, 2013).

Although the first pregnancy was reported in oocytes frozen using slow freezing in 1986, the application was limited to emergency medical indications since satisfactory success rates could not be achieved with this method. Another major limitation at that time was the lack of sufficient information on the long-term effects of the procedure. Slow freezing did not give effective results even in embryo freezing at the blastocyst stage, which has now been achieved with very high viability.

In slow freezing application, before the freezing stage, oocyte or embryos are gradually cooled by equilibration with low concentration CPAs (~10% v/v). With the decrease in temperature, the metabolism of the oocytes begins to slow down. Simultaneously, the concentration of CPAs is increased. This way tries to prevent the toxicity of CPAs and the formation of ice crystals. In this process, two important factors have a damaging effect: (i) Formation of intracellular ice crystals due to insufficient membrane permeability or unsuitable temperature during freezing and thawing; (ii) irreversible cell damage as a result of increased solute concentration called the "solution effect". While these two factors occur simultaneously, intracellular ice formation is active during rapid cooling and relatively slow rewarming, while the solution effect is active during slow freezing. As Luyet stated nearly 80 years ago, the formation of ice crystals is critical in the loss of viability of all cell types, and Luyet reported on an alternative approach called vitrification. The general principle in vitrification is to prevent ice crystal formation by transforming the fluid in and around the cell into a glassy amorphous solid with minimal water loss while the temperature drops rapidly.

3.6.1 Slow Freezing

In the slow freezing process, cell dehydration occurs gradually, and slow freezing temperatures are reached in a controlled manner with low CPA concentration treatment.

In the slow freezing process in which specially designed programmable freezing devices are used, the oocytes are first taken into solutions containing low concentration P-CPA (1.5 mol/L). Since the cell membrane is more permeable to water than CPAs, CPA does not change at the same level as the amount of intracellular water and cell shrinkage occurs. When an effective amount of CPA enters the cell, the cell re-expands and then the cell dehydration is re-stimulated by the addition of NP-CPA (mostly sucrose or trehalose ≤0.3 mol/L), creating an osmotic gradient. Oocytes are loaded into special straws and cooled to –8°C (–2°C/min) and manual seeding is performed at this stage to induce ice nucleation. In this way, the icing in the solution increases the dehydration and increases the extracellular solute concentration. The cooling continues slowly (–0.3°C/min to –1°C/min) and reaches –30°C. In this phase, the water in the solution is thoroughly removed and the amount of solute increases, reaching a state of amorphous solidification. When the temperature is reduced to –150°C (–50°C/min), the carriers are carefully immersed in liquid nitrogen at –196°C and taken to their special places in the storage tanks. The thawing process is performed quickly and in the opposite way to the stages during freezing. The cell is rehydrated by passing it through a gradient of decreasing concentrations of NP-CPA.

In the 1980s, when slow freezing applications were first on the agenda, DMSO was used as CPA and embryo freezing processes continued with a new protocol in which sugar was added. However, these studies based on clinical patient practice produced discouraging results because of low viability (50%), fertilisation (54%), and inadequate implantation and pregnancy success (10%).

3.6.2 Vitrification

Vitrification as a freezing technique ensures that oocytes are not exposed to physical damage associated with ice crystal formation during freezing, and high-density CPAs that form an amorphous glass during cooling are used. The newer 'vitrification' method has improved the success rate of post-thaw survival, fertilisation and implantation compared to slow freezing.

During the vitrification process, oocytes are prepared for freezing with high concentrations of CPAs and are frozen instantly and stored in tanks filled with liquid nitrogen at –196°C. Initially, in the equilibration phase, immediately after the oocytes are placed in the basic solution, they are kept in the gradually increased equilibration solution containing 7.5% ethylene glycol and 7.5% DMSO for a total of 5–15 minutes. Oocytes are then transferred to the vitrification solution containing 0.5 mol/L sucrose in addition to 15% ethylene glycol and 15% DMSO. After incubation for about 1 minute, they are transferred to special carriers with a minimal volume. Together, they are immersed in liquid nitrogen at –196°C, which has been sterilised by UV before to ensure direct contact. It is important to use a pipette tip with the appropriate diameter in the transfer stages of oocytes to prevent damage to the cell membrane. Sterilisation and suitability of the materials used increase the success of recovery. However, due to the high concentration of the solutions used, the toxicity potential is higher than with the slow freezing technique.

Permeable CPAs with low molecular weight such as DMSO and ethylene glycol displace water in the cell using osmotic pressure and prevent the formation of intracellular crystals without causing deformity in the cell. Increasing CPAs gradually increase the viability of oocytes while reducing the effect of osmotic shock and toxicity. DMSO and ethylene glycol lower the intracellular freezing temperature and form a glassy structure instead of ice crystals. Sucrose, one of the impermeable CPAs, provides the necessary osmotic exchange by balancing its extracellular concentration.

The thawing process is carried out quickly to prevent the formation of ice crystals. A carrier containing the cryopreserved oocyte is immersed in a water bath for closed vitrification and in a high sucrose concentration (1 mol/L) dissolving liquid for open vitrification. Afterwards, the removal of the CPAs is performed in the opposite way to the freezing process and the oocytes are stored in the appropriate culture medium.

In the slow freezing technique, low-concentration cryoprotectant solutions are used to cool at a very low rate ($0.3°C/min$). In vitrification, unlike slow cooling, cryopreservation is performed by rapid cooling ($2,500–30,000°C/min$) with dense cryoprotectant solutions. Programmable freezing devices with high investment costs are used in the slow freezing technique and the application period of the technique is quite long. While the cooling process takes about 15 minutes in the vitrification technique, this time can go up to 110 minutes in the slow freezing technique. In vitrification, the impact of the skill of the operator is greater than in slow freezing. Viability performance of oocytes using the vitrification technique, which requires operator experience and advanced manipulation skills, can be affected by inter-practitioner differences.

3.6.2.1 *Types of Oocyte Vitrification Carriers*

In the vitrification technique, the use of appropriate carriers, which are used for lossless and high-viability recovery of oocytes after thawing, plays an important role in success. In general, they are divided into two types: open and closed system vitrification carriers. Examples of open system vitrification carriers are unprotected Open Pulled Straw, Cryotech, Cryolock, Cryoleaf, and Vitri-Inga. These carriers allow the oocytes to come into direct contact with liquid nitrogen and generally allow very high rates of cooling. However, this method also has serious disadvantages. The liquid nitrogen in which the oocytes are stored is generally not sterile and can harbour many pathogens. In addition, the presence of some reactive chemical compounds in liquid nitrogen is high. On the other hand, CryoTip, High-Security Vitrification Straw, Cryopette, Rapid-i, VitriSafe and MicroSecure are among the closed system vitrification carrier types. They cannot achieve as effective a cooling rate as open system carriers, but they have the advantage that oocytes can be stored in complete isolation from the external environment and increase safety against dangerous effects that may occur during long-term storage (Vajta et al, 2015).

There have been publications that revealed a significant difference in oocyte viability rates between open and closed system carriers, and that viability and fertilisation rates are much higher in open systems. At that time, only De Munck's work showed that there was no difference between the viability rates of the two systems (De Munck et al, 2016). However, newer studies have demonstrated equal efficacy between open and closed systems (Gullo et al, 2020). According to a recent study conducted at S. Orsola-Malpighi University Hospital in Italy, no significant difference was observed in oocyte viability rates between open and closed system carriers. This study was carried out with the participation of 737 patients between 2015 and 2020. The patients were divided into two groups for vitrification using open and closed systems, and oocyte survival, fertilisation, division, pregnancy, implantation and miscarriage rates were compared between the two groups. Between these two groups, oocyte viability rate (70.3% vs. 73.3%), fertilisation rate (74.9% vs. 70.8%), division rate (90.6% vs. 90.3%), pregnancy/transfer rate (32.0%), implantation rate (19.9% vs. 19.9%) and miscarriage rates (22.1% vs. 21.5%) showed no statistically significant difference (Porcu et al, 2020).

Despite the successful use of open system carriers for vitrification, direct contact between sample and liquid nitrogen is not optimal due to the potential risk of cross-contamination between samples and accidental exposure to contaminants present in tanks. The use of closed system vitrification carriers eliminates these risks. Some reports confirm that although the temperature of liquid nitrogen is $-196.5°C$, it may contain microorganisms, bacteria and viruses that can cause infections. During long-term cryopreservation, the ice residue accumulated in storage poses a risk of microbial contamination to the stored samples. These ice crystals collect and trap other materials such as bacteria and fungal spores. In theory, stored samples could also be contaminated if liquid nitrogen and its vapours were contaminated; therefore, liquid nitrogen itself can be considered a potential source of pathogens during cryopreservation and long-term storage. This issue has raised serious concerns about the use of open devices in vitrification.

It has been hypothesised that testicular damage and "subsequent" infertility may occur following COVID-19 infection. In addition, sexual transmission of the disease has also been shown from the SARS-CoV-2 virus being detected in the sperm of infected patients. Hence, the risk of contamination has become a serious problem, especially for the COVID-19 outbreak and after. The results of current studies show that the high-security closed vitrification system is efficient and provides the most secure storage of biological samples, reducing the potential risk of viral contamination (Porcu et al, 2020). Therefore, the use of closed system carriers for the oocyte vitrification method is strongly recommended by the author of this chapter.

3.6.2.2 *Future Developments in Oocyte Vitrification*

Manual oocyte vitrification is a labour-intensive and time-consuming procedure. Embryologists continue to seek more standardised and highly successful techniques every day as they manage a stressful procedure that may involve cell loss during manipulation or due to a technical error. The recent emergence of robotic systems, which are called automated vitrification devices, is anticipated as an important start in reaching the inter-laboratory standard success rates of this technology, which has not yet become widespread.

The use of robotic systems for vitrification of mammalian embryos was first reported by Jun et al in 2015, promising higher viability and development rates compared to manual manipulation. In an article written by Sarah Lazarus in CNN Business in 2021, it was mentioned that cryo-robots will play an important role in preventing catastrophic loss of oocytes and embryos due to human errors. In 2018, it was stated that 4,000 oocytes were lost and incorrect embryo transfer was made in an IVF centre in Ohio, and that human errors could be eliminated with the development of automated storage and manipulation systems. In addition, the robot tanks used for the storage of frozen oocytes increase the success of cryopreservation by controlling the internal environment 17,000 times a day.

In contrast to cryopreservation of embryos, where serial usage over a few years until the desired family size is achieved is the norm, long-term storage of frozen oocytes is increasingly common especially if they were harvested for cancer patients. However, since cryo-robots are available in only a limited number of laboratories around the world, long-term application results and multicentre success rates are not yet known. The international laboratory accreditation and certification for oocyte freezing programs is not yet a requirement in many countries, and there are no specific international external accreditation programs. The need for global standardisation is increasing day by day, and banks that carry out oocyte freezing applications for donation need trans-national planning especially if 'export' is to be undertaken. The training of personnel and the monitoring of their performance are extremely important, and the use of electronic witnessing systems should be expanded to prevent human error. In many laboratories, the tracking of the tank maps is carried out manually and the cryo-tools on which the oocytes are loaded are handwritten. Labelling with special barcodes resistant to –196°C and using programs that provide tank tracking will play an active role in minimising human errors.

Apart from parameters such as age, weight, smoking and ethnicity, which are taken into account in donor selection in donation programs, testing for infectious diseases has become a standard procedure. In addition, taking family history and evaluating the risks in terms of hereditary genetic disease carriers and testing genetic conditions such as cystic fibrosis with a high carrier risk appear as routine criteria for donor selection. The concept of the "Certified Oocyte" has started to come to the fore especially in donation programs. In addition to many routine tests and evaluations performed on the donor, genetic examination in polar body cells means that each oocyte's chromosomes are numerically and structurally normal (euploid). Although genetic tests performed on polar body cells, where only maternal chromosome information can be accessed, is an approach that only a limited number of researchers have applied and its contribution to healthy birth rates is controversial, it is a precursor to genetic tests that can be performed on oocyte cells in the future.

References

De Munck N, Santos-Ribeiro S, Stoop D, Van de Velde H, Verheyen G. Open versus closed oocyte vitrification in an oocyte donation programme: a prospective randomized sibling oocyte study. Hum Reprod. 2016 Feb;31(2):377–84.

Donnez J, Dolmans MM. Fertility preservation in men and women: where are we in 2021? Are we rising to the challenge? Fertil Steril. 2021 May;115(5):1089–90.

Gullo G, Petousis S, Papatheodorou A, Panagiotidis Y, Margioula-Siarkou C, Prapas N, D'Anna R, Perino A, Cucinella G, Prapas Y. Closed vs. open oocyte vitrification methods are equally effective for blastocyst embryo transfers: prospective study from a sibling oocyte donation program. Gynecol Obstet Invest. 2020;85(2):206–12.

Porcu E, Tranquillo ML, Notarangelo L, Ciotti PM, Calza N, Zuffa S, Mori L, Nardi E, Dirodi M, Cipriani L, Labriola FS, Damiano G. High-security closed devices are efficient and safe to protect human oocytes from potential risk of viral contamination during vitrification and storage especially in the COVID-19 pandemic. J Assist Reprod Genet. 2021 Mar;38(3):681–8.

Practice Committees of the American Society for Reproductive Medicine and the Society for Assisted Reproductive Technology. Mature oocyte cryopreservation: a guideline. Fertil Steril. 2013 Jan;99(1):37–43.

Vajta G, Rienzi L, Ubaldi FM. Open versus closed systems for vitrification of human oocytes and embryos. Reprod Biomed Online. 2015 Apr;30(4):325–33.

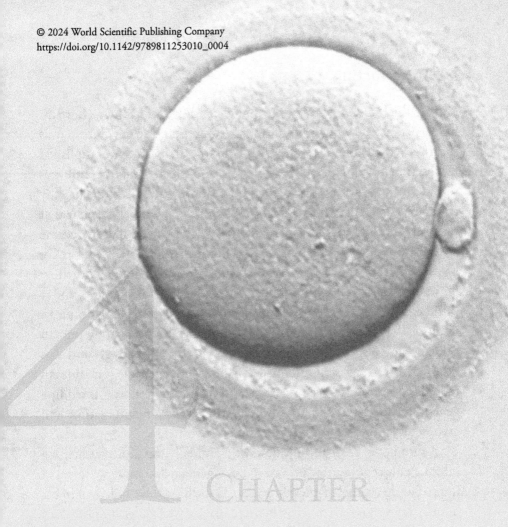

Alternatives to Oocyte Cryopreservation: Ovarian Cortex Freezing and *In Vitro* Maturation

Claus Yding Andersen

4.1 Introduction

During the last half-century, our understanding of fertility in humans has experienced a quantum leap. The reproductive revolution was spearheaded by Bob Edwards, who for the first time accomplished fertilisation of human oocytes *in vitro* and created unique embryos that were successfully used for procreation and birth of healthy children. His work, with contributions from many others, meant that for many infertile couples having their own biological children became a realistic opportunity. The sheer number of people who have benefitted from the *in vitro* fertilisation (IVF) technique since then illustrates the immense importance and impact of this method; today (ultimo 2023) we are approaching 12 million children being born as a result of IVF. It provided for the first time the ability to study human gametes and especially human oocytes in the laboratory and has resulted in a massive increase of new information on human reproduction, both basic science and clinically related, including genetic testing, nutritional requirements, *in vitro* manipulation and cryopreservation of both oocytes and embryos.

A number of these techniques, which initially was aimed at helping infertile couples, has now proved to be of general and more widespread interest and is being adapted in society as a whole. The ability to freeze human oocytes and embryos is a technique with huge implications beyond the group of infertile couples. This method allows suspended animation of oocytes and embryos in liquid nitrogen at −196°C. At this low temperature all biological processes are for all practical purposes stopped and the oocytes and embryos will remain viable, after thawing, decades after freezing and for all we know much longer. Thus, the method stops the clock with regard to ageing of oocytes and embryos with the implication that the age corresponds to the time of cryopreservation. The well-known *in vivo* deterioration of oocyte and embryo quality with increasing age accompanied with a reduced chance to conceive will not take place. At the time of thawing/ warming, the oocytes and embryos will possess a capacity for implantation corresponding to the age at which they were frozen and not to the biological age of the women attempting to conceive (provided they are not damaged by the freezing process itself).

Therefore, this method offers the possibility of postponing childbearing and still have available oocytes and/or embryos from a younger age. It allows timing of motherhood at the woman's own decision and basically provides women with the freedom to choose and plan their lives and careers in a new and fundamentally different way than earlier, when the biological clock and the reduced ability to conceive with age was an irrefutable fact of life. The method for cryopreservation was developed in response to the surplus oocytes and embryos generated from treating infertile couples with ovarian stimulation and IVF with the intention of increasing their chances of becoming pregnant, but has obviously far-reaching implications for society as a whole when used by women who are normally fertile. Often this group of women prefer to store unfertilised oocytes for fertility preservation because this leaves them with an option to decide who the biological father will be.

4.2 Advantages and Shortcomings of Current Practice of Freezing Oocytes

The method used for cryopreservation of oocytes — vitrification, which has now emerged as the standard technique — provides high survival rates and is the universally accepted method. In the best centres, survival rates exceeding 90% are not uncommon and the resulting embryos show almost identical implantation rates as freshly generated embryos (Cobo et al, 2015). Commercial media and methods are available, and it can be concluded that from a technical standpoint this is solved and has become the mainstream treatment.

However, the number of oocytes and their quality are highly variable and are important parameters for determining success with this technique — the more the better, and the better the quality the higher the chances of success (Sunkara et al, 2014). As the number of oocytes is determined during foetal life and constitutes the entire lifelong reproductive potential of a woman, the stock of oocytes and their quality becomes reduced with age, especially accelerating during the mid-thirties. Thus, the general rule for fertility preservation is that the younger the woman, the better the chances of a successful outcome.

Today fertility preservation of oocytes has been accomplished through two remarkable achievements in assisted reproduction. First, ovarian stimulation through administration of exogenous gonadotropins has proven to be capable of stimulating multiple follicles that result in a harvest of oocytes that roughly corresponds to the number of pre-ovulatory follicles developed. Thus, the normal one oocyte developed in connection with the natural menstrual cycle is now routinely greatly surpassed and ten or more oocytes are commonly collected (Sunkara et al, 2014). Secondly, these oocytes — or embryos if fertilised — can now be successfully cryopreserved through the developed vitrification methods that in the best case scenarios show survival rates of 90% or even more (Cobo et al, 2015). Depending on the number of follicles resulting from the ovarian stimulation protocol and the age of the woman, suspended animation of oocytes and the technical requirement for postponing childbearing is thus in place.

This scenario highlights two important lessons on human reproduction. First, it is not only the follicle, which in a natural cycle become the selected follicle and destined to undergo full development, and ovulate, that contains an oocyte with the full capacity to result in new offspring. Ovarian stimulation providing administration of exogenous gonadotropins secures growth and development of a number of follicles that are comparable to that of the natural cycle in terms of pregnancy potential of the enclosed oocytes. There are plenty of examples of four, five or more children from one round of ovarian stimulation. Taken together, the hormonal environment determines the health of follicles and the viability of the enclosed oocytes rather than the natural selection process itself governed by some as yet unknown mechanisms.

Ovarian stimulation targets the very last stages of follicular development. Right from activation of the resting follicles and until ovulation a period of four to six months will elapse, and the diameter will increase from around 40 μm to 20 mm. During this period the follicles are subjected to a number of different regulatory and intricate checkpoints and hormonal regulations, which are far from being fully understood. However, the developmental trajectory is characterised by a massive loss of follicles. In the reproductive younger years of a woman, it is estimated that around thousands or more follicles embark on growth during one month, but only one will make it to ovulation while the rest will undergo atresia. Thus, there is huge loss of follicles, accounting for more than 99% of all follicles present in the ovaries. We have now understood from ovarian stimulation that at least some of these follicles, which were destined to undergo atresia during the first part of the follicular phase in the natural menstrual cycle, can be saved and result in viable oocytes.

4.3 Freezing of Ovarian Tissue — Cryopreserving the Functional Unit of the Ovary

The ovarian pool of follicles is laid down during foetal life and constitutes the lifelong reproductive potential. The resting follicles are made up of primordial follicles with a small diameter of around 40 μm, which have not embarked on growth and development (Westergaard et al, 2007). This pool is sequentially recruited until it becomes exhausted around the time of menopause. The primordial follicles constitute, at any moment in time in any woman's life, more than 90% of all follicles present in the ovaries. This clearly demonstrates that the biggest potential for fertility preservation is the resting follicles as they represent by far the most plentiful source of oocytes, provided methods to use the oocytes for reproduction can be developed.

Furthermore, anatomically the primordial follicles are specifically located next to the cortex region — just one to two millimetres below the surface of the ovary (Figure 4.1). This anatomical feature of the human ovary facilitates cryopreservation of the isolated cortex in a thickness of one to two millimetres with its almost entire content of primordial follicles. Thus, the functional unit of the ovary, the follicle, is preserved and explains why transplanted frozen/thawed ovarian

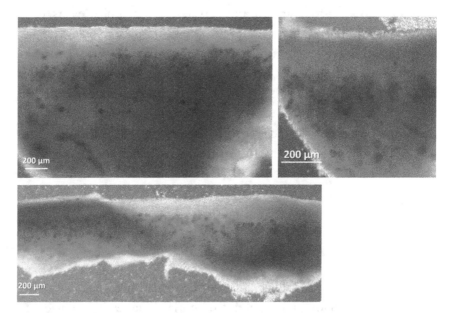

Figure 4.1 Three different examples of human ovarian cortex with viable primordial follicles stained red with Neutral Red. Below the ovarian surface epithelium, the abundance of follicles makes it attractive for fertility preservation. Research and development needs to optimise the quality of the oocytes resulting from this tissue to provide improved clinical results.

tissue can re-establish an ovarian organ function, since each of the primordial follicles has the potential to grow to the pre-ovulatory stage and concomitantly secrete hormones including sex steroids to ensure proper conditions for the development of a conceptus. Surprisingly, therefore, the ovary is currently the only human organ that sustains freezing and maintains an organ function upon transplantation. There have now been methods developed that tolerate freezing of this type of follicles with very high efficiency — around 90% survival rate (Kristensen et al, 2018). Retrieval of the tissue is performed through a minor operation in which either part of the ovarian tissue is excised or one of the two ovaries. The tissue needs to be prepared for cryopreservation in a laboratory and is during this process cut into a number of small pieces (5 × 5 mm) (Figure 4.2), which are frozen and stored in separate ampoules in liquid nitrogen (Andersen et al, 2012; Andersen et al, 2019). This allows for an individual approach in thawing out the number of pieces of cortex that is considered appropriate for the individual woman.

In essence the technical side of this method is at an acceptable level; however, overall, the transplantation methods and their effectiveness are still far from being sufficiently developed for this method. Follicle loss in connection with transplantation is massive, which limits its efficacy and the functional lifespan of the transplanted tissue (Figure 4.2).

It is estimated that around 200 children have currently been born from replacement of frozen thawed ovarian tissue, which clearly indicates that it is early days with a lot of optimisation to take place in order to increase efficacy. In most cases the indications for performing the procedure are patients suffering from a disease where proper treatment poses a risk of destroying all the follicles (e.g., cancer) or where the disease itself causes demise of follicles (e.g., Turner syndrome patients) (Dolmans et al, 2021). Thus, these techniques have not yet found a place for fertility preservation in healthy women who want to postpone reproduction.

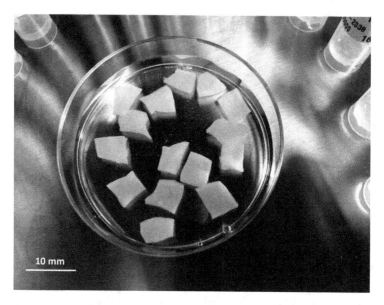

Figure 4.2 Frozen/thawed human ovarian cortex ready to be transplanted to the woman from where it originated, representing around 50% of one whole ovary. Each piece of cortex is separately frozen in individual ampoules and contains a large number of resting follicles depending on the age of the woman. After transplantation the tissue will be revascularised and the resting follicles will start to grow and eventually develop into pre-ovulatory follicles ready to undergo ovulation and release a mature oocyte and provide fertility. The development of follicles will provide the woman with menstrual cycles and circulating levels of sex steroids and other hormones irrespective of her age. Further, these pieces of ovarian cortex may be subjected to *in vitro* follicle activation before transplantation and is likely to result in an increased development of follicles shortly after transplantation, which may provide a window for increased fertility.

The efficacy by which transplantation of ovarian tissue restores fertility has recently been addressed by a publication involving five major European centres, which have pooled their data (Dolmans et al, 2021). From a total of 285 women who had frozen/thawed ovarian tissue transplanted, one in four succeeded in having a child. A single important factor for success was age, and those who conceived were up to five years younger than those who failed ($p < 0.001$).

However, the outcome of IVF treatment in these women are far from being comparable with standard results from IVF. The number of oocytes retrieved after ovarian stimulation is only a fraction of what is normally observed. Furthermore, embryo development is poor resulting in only 50% of patients having embryo transfer, in spite of repeated attempts at ovarian stimulation in many cases. Of those who did undergo embryo transfer, 43% succeeded in having a child. The small number of oocytes retrieved during IVF clearly demonstrates that the number of surviving follicles is severely reduced and that these patients behave as poor responders. This highlights that new methods need to be developed to increase follicle survival rate.

It is obviously of interest to compare the efficacy in terms of conception after utilisation of frozen oocytes as related to ovarian tissue. A comparison is not yet available for healthy women who wish to postpone reproduction, but attempts have been made for patients who suffered from a malignant disease at the time of fertility preservation. In a study from 2018, the Spanish IVI group reported from two relatively large groups of patients either receiving fertility preservation by freezing mature oocytes after ovarian stimulation (N = 1024) or by having ovarian cortical tissue frozen (N = 800) (Diaz-Garcia et al, 2018). The study included 49 patients who returned for collection of oocytes, whereas 44 patients requested transplantation of ovarian tissue. They reported that 16 women had a child after using their vitrified oocytes and 10 patients obtained a child after having tissue transplanted (of which five required IVF). The conclusion was that although no statistical difference was found between the two groups, it appeared that oocyte vitrification was more effective than ovarian tissue freezing. However, these two groups were not compared on an intention-to-treat basis, which would be the correct way to compare the two groups. In the oocyte vitrification group only patients who actually had oocytes retrieved were included, whereas the ovarian tissue freezing group included patients in whom the tissue did not start to work after transplantation, so failures of collecting oocytes were excluded in the oocyte freezing group but included in the ovarian tissue freezing group. Furthermore, the study included patients where the observation period was only five months after transplantation, which is too short a period, since the ovarian tissue has barely started to work after five months and this is too early for the tissue to support a pregnancy. For instance, women may conceive five years after being transplanted with ovarian tissue, which was beyond the average observation time in the IVI study, and only at that point will they change group from failures to successes. Both these circumstances will make the two groups more similar and it is likely that overall efficacy is quite similar between the two methods. This is

Table 4.1 Advantages and disadvantages of fertility preservation by freezing of ovarian tissue.

Advantages	Disadvantages
Cryopreserves the follicle — the hormone-producing functional unit of the ovary	Requires an operation to excise and potentially replace ovarian tissue
Freezes the pool of primordial follicles — by far the most abundant follicle type in any ovary	Transplantation is very ineffective with massive follicle loss
Allows *in vitro* follicle activation prior to transplantation or any future development to more efficiently utilise the available follicles and oocytes	May require an IVF procedure to conceive
In case the tissue is not needed for reproduction, it may be used for securing endocrine production of sex steroids if needed	Efficacy needs to be improved
Allows natural conception after transplantation	May be more costly than oocyte freezing
May be combined with IVM using oocytes from small antral follicles	

notable especially given that the IVI group is renowned for its fine results with oocyte vitrification.

Taken together, ovarian tissue freezing is a relatively new technique that has not yet been fully developed. It has the advantage of targeting the most abundant type of follicles, and provided that this type of follicles can grow and develop into a resulting higher number of mature oocytes that can be used for procreation after appropriate maturation either *in vitro* or *in vivo,* this method has the potential to become the ultimate goal and the most preferred method for fertility preservation in the future. However, currently a lot more research and development of this whole concept is needed for it to become a clear choice over freezing of mature oocytes.

4.4 Utilisation of Oocytes from Earlier Stages of Follicular Development — Introducing *In Vitro* Maturation of Oocytes

Follicle growth and development is a continuous selection process with follicles entering atresia at all stages of progression from the time the primordial follicle leaves the dormant pool until the chosen pre-ovulatory follicle prepares to undergo ovulation. Whereas the tangible result of ovarian tissue freezing is the plentiful resting follicle pool, freezing of mature oocytes are at the other end of follicle development right before ovulation, where the pool of follicles has been subjected to the selection and atresia rate naturally occurring all the way until ovarian stimulation is commenced. However, it is now possible to access immature oocytes collected from small antral follicles en route in the growth and development process to become a fully mature follicle. Thus, these types of oocytes are likely to be more available in higher numbers than those collected at the fully mature state just before ovulation. Provided they receive *in vitro* maturation (IVM) that allows for clinical use with an acceptable success, this is yet another alternative to conventional freezing of *in vivo* matured oocytes collected at oocyte pick-up in conjunction with ovarian stimulation (Telfer and Andersen, 2021).

Ovarian tissue freezing has allowed the development and optimisation of IVM on human oocytes, because often one whole ovary is excised for fertility preservation with only the cortical tissue undergoing freezing, while the surplus medulla is discharged with its content of growing follicles (Cadenas et al, 2021). Thus, this method takes advantage of the *in vivo* growth of follicles to essentially bypass the difficult and complex first steps in human folliculogenesis at the expense of some follicles loss due to atresia, and then collect oocytes from follicles with a diameter of just a few millimetres, taking advantage of the reduced number and atresia rate compared to collecting oocytes in the pre-ovulatory stage. Whereas excising one whole ovary for fertility preservation for non-medical indications is seldom an option, this limits this procedure to those oocytes that can be aspirated from small antral follicles from non-stimulated ovaries, which currently reduces the number of immature oocytes that can be collected. However, a number of clinicians are now developing the field of oocyte aspiration from small antral follicles *in situ* and combining that with IVM (Sonigo et al, 2020). While this approach needs a lot of development and improvement for both the collection of oocytes and the IVM procedure, it has the advantage of no ovarian stimulation with exogenous hormones being required and may be repeated at relatively short intervals when a new cohort of small antral follicles has been developed in the ovaries. This allows for multiple collections of oocytes at a relatively low cost and may in this way boost the number of oocytes that can be used for fertility preservation and freezing. Women with polycystic ovary syndrome were the first group of women to whom this method was applied because these women present with an augmented pool of small antral follicles from which immature oocytes may be collected (Sonigo et al, 2020). Indeed, more than 100 immature oocytes have been collected from one ovary retrieved for fertility preservation from women with polycystic ovary syndrome (Nikiforov et al, 2020).

It now appears that cumulus oocyte complexes from these small antral follicles possess characteristics that are attractive to exploit in connection with IVM. The follicle-stimulating hormone (FSH) receptor expression on cumulus cells from small antral follicles is noticeably increased compared to later on in follicular development (Cadenas et al, 2021). Therefore, the responsivity towards FSH stimulation is probably augmented and by exposing the cumulus oocyte complexes to high levels of FSH, an accelerated maturation process is induced, which therefore bypasses the atresia. This has previously been observed by Gougeon (1996), who reported the atresia rate of human follicles at different developmental stages and found that follicles with diameters from 0.9–2 millimetres had an atresia rate of 15–24%, while follicles from 2–8 millimetres had an atresia rate of 55–77%, which may reflect that the FSH receptor expression was dramatically reduced during these developmental stages.

Taken together, human IVM is currently undergoing improvements based on the use of oocytes from small antral follicles and is likely to constitute an important alternative for fertility preservation by freeing mature oocytes in the future.

4.5 *In Vitro* Follicle Activation — Exciting Outlook but not yet a Clinical Procedure

Activation of growth in resting follicles has been achieved with good success especially in rodent species (Reddy et al, 2008; Adhikari et al, 2009; Li et al, 2010). It has been shown that follicle activation is critically dependent on the phosphatidylinositol-3′-kinase signalling pathway (Li et al, 2010; McLaughlin et al, 2014; Grosbois & Demeestere, 2018; Kallen et al, 2018; Maidarti et al, 2020). An important component of this pathway is the phosphatase and tensin homolog deleted on chromosome ten (PTEN), which attenuates and acts as a negative regulator of initiation of follicle growth (Reddy et al, 2008; Maidarti et al, 2020; review: Zhao et al, 2021). If the action of PTEN is removed or downregulated from the ovaries — either in knockout mouse models or by using pharmacological inhibitors *in vitro* — it is possible to activate follicular growth in both humans and animals (Kawamura et al, 2013; Suzuki et al, 2015; Zhai et al, 2016; review: Zhao et al, 2021).

However, studies in humans have been less consistent with only small clinical studies showing marginal effects, if at all, on *in vitro* follicle activation and improvement of clinical results (Lunding et al, 2020; Ferreri et al, 2020; Kawamura et al, 2020). It appears that despite increased understanding of the molecular mechanisms governing follicular activation, translation into clinically applicable methods still requires development and the concept is currently receiving less attention both clinically and in the laboratory.

Nevertheless, a continued research effort is likely to result in a method to achieve follicle activation as well for human ovarian tissue. Provided that a clinically acceptable method for follicle activation is developed, it will be of interest to the relatively large group of women undergoing fertility preservation at an advanced reproductive age. The cortex contains a high number of resting follicles even in reproductive-age women and provided that these follicles can be activated *in vitro* and then transplanted, it is hypothesised that a relatively large cohort of follicles can be recruited for pre-ovulatory follicle development after four to eight months — perhaps after appropriate stimulation with exogenous hormones. Tentatively this increased activation of a fraction of the resting follicles should result in a larger cohort of growing follicles and lead to harvest of more mature oocytes suitable for procreation, thereby resulting in better chances for a pregnancy than conventional ovarian stimulation regimes. Theoretically, such a procedure is founded on the abundant pool of resting follicles combined with an activation step leading to utilisation of a much larger fraction of follicles/oocytes than conventional ovarian stimulation regimes.

4.6 Conclusion and Forward Perspectives

As a general trend in society and in parallel with more women becoming well educated and pursuing careers, more and more women postpone childbearing. As a result, more women experience difficulties in conceiving because age and reproduction work in opposite directions, especially in terms of quantity and quality of the available oocytes. The problem of many reproductive-age women is basically: too few eggs and too old eggs to endure good chances of pregnancies. This is already a sizeable problem to many women in different parts of the world, particularly in the US where companies now embark on helping their staff achieving fertility preservation. The method of ovarian stimulation and collection of mature oocytes developed in connection with treatment of infertile women has now been applied to the group of women who seek fertility preservation due to anxiety of the effect of age on their reproductive possibilities.

Alternative methods for fertility preservation that focus on earlier stages of follicular development are now becoming of interest for research and development. Follicles in earlier stages of follicular development are more abundant and can now be cryopreserved with good efficacy. The developmental capacity of these follicles is not yet determined but a lot better than anticipated, and research now focuses on providing strategies to obtain mature oocytes suitable for procreation in higher numbers and with better quality than the conventional ovarian stimulation strategies. These strategies include better survival upon transplantation of frozen/thawed ovarian tissue potentially combined with *in vitro* follicle activation prior to transplantation and utilising immature oocytes from small antral follicles. Thus, the key is understanding human folliculogenesis a lot better, especially during the earlier stages of follicular development.

It is, however, important to point out that these new methods are under development and do not currently guarantee success rates greater than ovarian stimulation and oocyte vitrification. Indeed, the effect of age is still a determining factor for success but approaches to obtain more oocytes of better quality than the current technologies can provide is a likely scenario in the coming years.

Thus, the reproductive revolution initiated by Bod Edwards is far from being over, and there is still much research to be done into the intricate and complicated processes leading to successful procreation. This knowledge will help women who wish to postpone childbearing experience improved chances of having their own biological children and will provide more choices to women in connection with reproduction.

References

Adhikari D, Zheng W, Shen Y, Gorre N, Hämäläinen T, Cooney AJ, Huhtaniemi I, Lan ZJ, Liu K. Tsc/mTORC1 signaling in oocytes governs the quiescence and activation of primordial follicles. Hum Mol Genet. 2010 Feb 1;19(3):397–410.

Andersen CY, Kristensen SG, Greve T, Schmidt KT. Cryopreservation of ovarian tissue for fertility preservation in young female oncological patients. Future Oncol. 2012;8:595–608.

Andersen CY, Mamsen LS, Kristensen SG. Freezing of ovarian tissue and clinical opportunities. Reproduction. 2019;158:F27–F34.

Cadenas J, Nikiforov D, Pors SE, Zuniga LA, Wakimoto Y, Ghezelayagh Z, Mamsen LS, Kristensen SG, Andersen CY. A threshold concentration of FSH is needed during IVM of ex vivo collected human oocytes. J Assist Reprod Genet. 2021;38:1341–8.

Cobo A, Garrido N, Pellicer A, Remohí J. Six years' experience in ovum donation using vitrified oocytes: Report of cumulative outcomes, impact of storage time, and development of a predictive model for oocyte survival rate. Fertil Steril. 2015 Dec;104(6):1426–34.e1–8.

Diaz-Garcia C, Domingo J, Garcia-Velasco JA, Herraiz S, Mirabet V, Iniesta I, Cobo A, Remohí J, Pellicer A. Oocyte vitrification versus ovarian cortex transplantation in fertility preservation for adult women undergoing gonadotoxic treatments: A prospective cohort study. Fertil Steril. 2018;109:478–85.

Dolmans MM, von Wolff M, Poirot C, Diaz-Garcia C, Cacciottola L, Boissel N, Liebenthron J, Pellicer A, Donnez J, Andersen CY. Transplantation of cryopreserved ovarian tissue in a series of 285 women: A review of five leading European centers. Fertil Steril. 2021;115:1102–15.

Ferreri J, Fàbregues F, Calafell JM, Solernou R, Borrás A, Saco A, Manau D, Carmona F. Drug-free in-vitro activation of follicles and fresh tissue autotransplantation as a therapeutic option in patients with primary ovarian insufficiency. Reprod Biomed Online. 2020 Feb;40(2):254–60.

Gougeon A. Regulation of ovarian follicular development in primates: Facts and hypotheses. Endocr Rev. 1996;17:121–55.

Grosbois J, Demeestere I. Dynamics of PI3K and Hippo signaling pathways during in vitro human follicle activation. Hum Reprod. 2018;33:1705–14.

Kallen A, Polotsky AJ, Johnson J. Untapped reserves: Controlling primordial follicle growth activation. Trends Mol Med. 2018;24:319–31.

Kawamura K, Cheng Y, Suzuki N, Deguchi M, Sato Y, Takae S et al. Hippo signaling disruption and Akt stimulation of ovarian follicles for infertility treatment. Proc Natl Acad Sci U S A. 2013;110:17474–9.

Kawamura K, Ishizuka B, Hsueh AJW. Drug-free in-vitro activation of follicles for infertility treatment in poor ovarian response patients with decreased ovarian reserve. Reprod Biomed Online. 2020 Feb;40(2):245–253.

Kristensen SG, Liu Q, Mamsen LS, Greve T, Pors SE, Bjørn AB, Ernst E, Macklon KT, Andersen CY. A simple method to quantify follicle survival in cryopreserved human ovarian tissue. Hum Reprod. 2018 Dec 1;33(12):2276–84.

Li J, Kawamura K, Cheng Y, Liu S, Klein C, Liu S et al. Activation of dormant ovarian follicles to generate mature eggs. Proc Natl Acad Sci U S A. 2010;107:10280–4.

Lunding SA, Andersen AN, Hardardottir L, Olesen H, Kristensen SG, Andersen CY et al. Hippo signaling, actin polymerization, and follicle activation in fragmented human ovarian cortex. Mol Reprod Dev. 2020;87:711–9.

Maidarti M, Anderson RA, Telfer EE. Crosstalk between PTEN/PI3K/Akt signalling and DNA damage in the oocyte: Implications for primordial follicle activation, oocyte quality and ageing. Cells. 2020 Jan 14;9(1):200.

McLaughlin M, Kinnell HL, Anderson RA, Telfer EE. Inhibition of phosphatase and tensin homologue (PTEN) in human ovary in vitro results in increased activation of primordial follicles but compromises development of growing follicles. Mol Hum Reprod. 2014;20:736–44.

Nikiforov D, Junping C, Cadenas J, Shukla V, Blanshard R, Pors SE, Kristensen SG, Macklon KT, Colmorn L, Ernst E, Bay-Bjørn AM, Ghezelayagh Z, Wakimoto Y, Grøndahl ML, Hoffmann E, Andersen CY. Improving the maturation rate of human oocytes collected ex vivo during the cryopreservation of ovarian tissue. J Assist Reprod Genet. 2020;37:891–904.

Reddy P, Liu L, Adhikari D, Jagarlamudi K, Rajareddy S, Shen Y et al. Oocyte-specific deletion of Pten causes premature activation of the primordial follicle pool. Science. 2008;319:611–3.

Sonigo C, Bajeux J, Boubaya M, Eustache F, Sifer C, Lévy V, Grynberg M, Sermondade N. In vitro maturation is a viable option for urgent fertility preservation in young women with hematological conditions. Hematol Oncol. 2020;38:560–4.

Sunkara SK, Khalaf Y, Maheshwari A, Seed P, Coomarasamy A. Association between response to ovarian stimulation and miscarriage following IVF: An analysis of 124 351 IVF pregnancies. Hum Reprod. 2014 Jun;29(6):1218–24.

Suzuki N, Yoshioka N, Takae S, Sugishita Y, Tamura M, Hashimoto S et al. Successful fertility preservation following ovarian tissue vitrification in patients with primary ovarian insufficiency. Hum Reprod. 2015;30:608–15.

Telfer EE, Andersen CY. In vitro growth and maturation of primordial follicles and immature oocytes. Fertil Steril. 2021;115:1116–25.

Westergaard CG, Byskov AG, Andersen CY. Morphometric characteristics of the primordial to primary follicle transition in the human ovary in relation to age. Hum Reprod. 2007;22:2225–31.

Zhai J, Yao G, Dong F, Bu Z, Cheng Y, Sato Y, Hu L, Zhang Y, Wang J, Dai S et al. In vitro activation of follicles and fresh tissue auto-transplantation in primary ovarian insufficiency patients. J Clin Endocrinol Metab. 2016;101:4405–12.

Zhao Y, Feng H, Zhang Y, Zhang JV, Wang X, Liu D, Wang T, Li RHW, Ng EHY, Yeung WSB, Rodriguez-Wallberg KA, Liu K. Current understandings of core pathways for the activation of mammalian primordial follicles. Cells. 2021 Jun 13;10(6):1491.

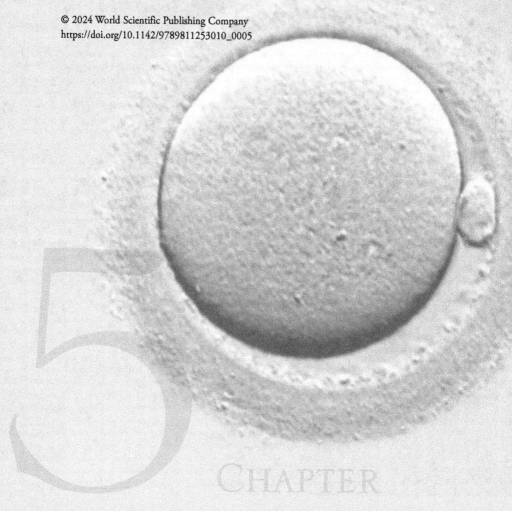

CHAPTER

Worldwide Trends in Oocyte Cryopreservation; Maternal and Neonatal Outcomes Following Oocyte Cryopreservation

Abey Eapen

Since the invention of assisted reproductive technology (ART) treatments, several key adjunct procedures have been added at timely intervals. Although many of these techniques were introduced on an experimental basis and eventually lost their "glamour", oocyte cryopreservation is a technique that stood the test of time. Freezing of human germ cells or tissues plays an essential role in providing reproductive autonomy and empowerment for persons interested in preserving their future fertility potential. Oocyte cryopreservation was accepted as an ethically permissible ART technique in the last decade.

The average maternal age at the time of first pregnancy has steadily increased since the 1970s. The Organization for Economic Co-operation and Development data demonstrated an increase of 2–5 years in the average age of women at childbirth between 1970 and 2015. The age of the oocyte source remains the primary determinant of the chances of a live birth. Women are therefore faced with fertility challenges. Even though initially more prevalent in developed countries, this is a trend that is now identified worldwide. Globally, the delay in childbearing has been attributed to better access to education, increasing demands in education and professional goals, relationship issues, and societal and other personal reasons. Combined with the age-related decline in ovarian reserve and oocyte quality, the trend of delaying motherhood has resulted in much debate for an increase in demand and need for oocyte cryopreservation.

There are several interchangeable terms like social egg freezing, elective egg freezing, fertility preservation, and oocyte banking for anticipated gamete exhaustion (AGE banking) used to indicate oocyte cryopreservation. There are also possible disparities in access to this technique as financial funding for non-medical oocyte cryopreservation is limited. Furthermore, some countries have legislative restrictions on this technique for non-medical indications. It is well known that persons who undergo oocyte cryopreservation are commonly Caucasians, highly educated or middle-class professionals in their mid to late thirties.

Although the first live birth resulting from *in vitro* fertilisation (IVF) using a frozen oocyte occurred in the mid-1980s, a significant breakthrough relating to oocyte cryopreservation happened only over the last decade with the introduction of 'ultra-rapid' freezing in liquid nitrogen, more widely known as the 'vitrification technique'. Studies have suggested that the addition of vitrification in the oocyte cryopreservation technique improved oocyte survival, fertilisation rates, embryo cleavage rates, and availability of embryos of superior quality when compared to the slow freezing technique. A recent International Federation of Fertility Societies' report (2019) shows that egg freezing is being performed in over half of 82 countries surveyed. Most clinics perform both medical and non-medical oocyte cryopreservation procedures.

In December 2009, the Israel National Bioethics Council issued recommendations permitting egg freezing for medical and non-medical indications. With improvements in technology matched by clinical outcomes, the European Society for Human Reproduction and Embryologists (ESHRE) in 2012 issued guidance for all stakeholders approving the use of planned oocyte cryopreservation. The American Society of Reproductive Medicine (ASRM) and the Society for Assisted Reproductive Technology (SART) announced in 2013 to no longer consider oocyte cryopreservation an experimental technique, even though they do not recommend it for age-related decline in fertility. Further, in 2014, Canadian Fertility and Andrology society also approved oocyte cryopreservation.

Despite emerging techniques like ovarian tissue cryopreservation and *in vitro* maturation gaining more interest, oocyte cryopreservation is the most established, safe, and cost-effective option. This has led to employer-sponsored elective oocyte cryopreservation, e.g., in the United States, where major technology companies (Apple, Google, and Facebook) provide their employees with more options to time and plan their fertility aspirations.

The Human Oocyte Preservation Experience registry data confirm better clinical pregnancy rates and live birth rates with donor oocytes than autologous oocytes. Therefore, the age at the time of retrieval, the number of cycles needed to achieve an optimal number, and the age at which these oocytes are used for treatment are important factors determining the cumulative chances of pregnancy following oocyte cryopreservation. As a general rule, it is ideal to undergo oocyte cryopreservation at an earlier age. The value of this technique is minimal in persons under the age of 30 and those over 41 years of age. The trend of oocyte cryopreservation cycles continues to rise on a year-by-year basis; however, the projected success rates for chances of a pregnancy after oocyte cryopreservation are based on a very low number of studies. Most data relating to success rates following oocyte cryopreservation are from internal unpublished data or clinic-specific data based on small numbers.

With the availability of easy, one-stop biomarker assessment of ovarian reserve testing and the possible diagnosis of diminished ovarian reserve, as well as patient-friendly online 'egg freezing calculators', there is significant public awareness and media attention towards oocyte cryopreservation technique. Several high-quality studies have demonstrated that diminished ovarian reserve is not associated with infertility. Therefore, it is imperative that persons planning oocyte cryopreservation for non-medical indications be provided psychological support and ethical, evidence-based, and transparent medical advice to narrow the knowledge gap in 'under' and 'over' estimation of the individual's reproductive potential.

There is a wide range of indications for oocyte cryopreservation, including medical and non-medical reasons, as discussed in Table 5.1.

5.1 Considerations Prior to Oocyte Cryopreservation

With imminent health implications, patients have a short timeframe to initiate lifesaving chemoradiation from the cancer diagnosis. According to the latest guidelines, all oncology medical professionals

Table 5.1   Indications for oocyte freezing.

Medical Indications	(a) Cancers which may result in potential sterilising chemoradiotherapy
	(b) Benign conditions needing ovarian surgery (e.g., borderline ovarian tumours), impending ovarian failure, or a personal history of diminished ovarian reserve or severe endometriosis
	(c) Systemic diseases needing initiation of long-term chemotherapy (e.g., the use of long-term methotrexate in a woman with a history of systemic lupus erythematosus)
	(d) Family member freezing oocytes for their offspring with a sex chromosome abnormality (e.g., mother freezing oocytes for an offspring with Turner's syndrome)
	(e) Prior to gender reaffirmation surgery
Non-medical Indications	(a) Advancing maternal age
	(b) Delaying pregnancy due to relationship status, goals in career, or education
	(c) Unanticipated relationship issues while undergoing IVF treatment
	(d) As part of 'donation' and 'sharing' IVF program followed by some IVF clinics
	(e) Lack of availability of sperm on the day of egg retrieval
	(f) Religious objections on creating supernumerary embryos
	(g) Other social aspects relating to financial stability or better home environment for their offspring

are encouraged to refer patients for a fertility preservation consultation, ideally to a centre with facilities to cryopreserve gametes/tissue. With emerging alternative options (e.g., ovarian cortex preservation), some oncologists are sceptical about delaying chemoradiation for ovarian stimulation (particularly for young females with an excellent prognosis for survival following chemotherapy or those with significantly advanced cancer staging). These patients, along with the emotional stress associated with the disease per se, are also faced with time constraints and significant costs associated with controlled ovarian stimulation for oocyte retrieval and cryopreservation.

On the other hand, oocyte cryopreservation for social indications faces some other challenges. There is a lack of agreement regarding the optimal timing for oocyte cryopreservation. The age of the female partner undergoing ovarian stimulation is the single factor determining the outcome of IVF treatment. Several observational cohort studies suggest that even though it is ideal to undergo oocyte cryopreservation under 35 years, live birth rates remain stable until about 36 to 38 years. While the number of cryopreserved oocytes is also important, a retrospective observational multicentre study suggested that the live birth rates were higher in women under the age of 35, compared to those over 36 years, despite utilising a similar number of oocytes (Johnston et al, 2021).

The recommendations for the individual patient must be specific to their family-building goals and recognise the risk of declining future fertility.

5.2 Ooocyte Cryopreservation Around the World

5.2.1 The Experience of Oocyte Cryopreservation in the United Kingdom

Over the last decade in the United Kingdom, oocyte cryopreservation cycles have increased tenfold, from just under 230 cycles in 2009 to almost 2,400 cycles in 2019. The data was published by the Human Fertilization and Embryology Authority in 2018 for 2014–2016. In 2016, 32% of women undergoing oocyte cryopreservation were under 35, and 62% were under the age of 38. A total of 1,173 oocyte cryopreservation cycles and 519 oocyte thaw cycles resulted in a live birth rate of 19% per embryo transfer, compared to 21% for fresh IVF treatment. However, this data did not distinguish between women undergoing IVF using frozen donor oocytes and women undergoing IVF using autologous frozen oocytes.

A cross-sectional survey conducted in the United Kingdom assessed the motivations and perceptions of women who underwent social oocyte cryopreservation for ten years since 2008. The study demonstrated that despite the physical, financial, and psychological burdens, only a small minority of women experienced regret after oocyte cryopreservation for non-medical reasons. Based on this trend, it is anticipated that it is likely that demand for egg freezing will continue to increase.

The Royal College of Obstetricians and Gynaecologists opines that elective oocyte cryopreservation proved an opportunity to 'mitigate the inevitable decline in fertility' due to advancing age. The College also calls for counselling risks related to procedural and financial aspects, and highlights the need to improve public education about the age-related decline in female infertility.

A retrospective cohort study of 167 women who had 184 social egg freezing cycles at an inner city IVF Unit in London between 2016 and 2022 was undertaken (Kakkar et al, 2023). The mean age at egg freezing was 37.1 years and the mean number of eggs obtained per retrieval was 9.5, with highest mean number frozen for women under 35. Some 16% of women returned to use their frozen eggs during the study period with an average freezing duration of 3.9 years, and 23 embryo transfers were carried out in 20 women. Crucial determinants of outcome were the age of the woman at time of freeze and the number of eggs thawed. Irrespective of the age of the woman, if more than 15 eggs were thawed the live birth rate was 45% per patient compared to 13% where less than 15 eggs were available to thaw.

5.2.2 The Experience of Oocyte Cryopreservation in the Rest of Europe

One in ten couples in Europe is affected by infertility. Europe currently has the lowest fertility rate globally, with women on average having

1.58 children each in 2014, far below the rate of 2.1 needed to maintain the population at current levels. A survey analysing responses to views on fertility treatments (*Listening in: IVF and Fertility in Europe [LIFE]*) from over 6,000 men and women in France, Germany, Italy, Spain, Sweden, and the United Kingdom suggested 60% of respondents were in favour of egg freezing for lifestyle reasons, such as starting a family later in life.

In Italy, the fertility rate remains below 1.5, and the average maternal age has increased over the last 20 years. Italy thus has the lowest fertility rates in Europe. A survey of 930 female students at the University of Padova (Italy) assessed their knowledge and attitudes on social egg freezing in 2019. The study suggested that while 34.3% of the students were aware of oocyte cryopreservation procedures for non-medical indications, only 19.5% favoured social egg freezing (Tazzo et al, 2019).

A recent study analysed data from the annual reports of the National Registry of Medically Assisted Reproduction and the Italian Statistical Institute from 2015 to 2018. As Italy relies on foreign egg banks for oocyte donation treatment, the study calls for an urgent need to encourage planned oocyte cryopreservation (preferably before the age of 40) and the need to establish a national biobank and specific regulation for gamete donation.

In Spain, recent studies have suggested a significant difference in survival and clinical outcomes after oocyte vitrification based on indications for cryopreservation. There was a 26% difference in live birth rates in those diagnosed with cancer compared to women who underwent elective oocyte freezing in age-matched groups. A difference was observed when outcomes were compared in women with endometriosis and those who had elective oocyte cryopreservation. There was a difference of 6% in oocyte survival rate, 16% in implantation rate, and 6.9% in live birth rate when comparing women with endometriosis to women undergoing elective oocyte freezing. Studies suggest that age, patient prognosis, and the number of oocytes should be evaluated while assessing the outcome of oocyte cryopreservation technique (Cobo et al, 2021).

Elective oocyte freezing has been offered in Sweden for more than ten years. The utilisation rate is similar to other countries in Europe. A follow-up study of a subset (254 women) who electively vitrified oocytes at a private IVF clinic was conducted between 2011 and 2017. 38 women returned for autologous IVF treatment cycle with a mean age of 36.9 (range 23 to 43) at the time of oocyte cryopreservation. The cumulative live birth rates were 63%, 26%, and 0% in women of ages 36–37, 38–39, and 40 years of age at the time of vitrification, respectively (Wennberg, 2019).

Health professionals in Europe have set up collaborative efforts to educate professionals and collect data for outcomes for oocyte cryopreservation. Some examples include the Danish Network (www. rigshopitlet.dk), which is a centralised network for the practical implementation of fertility-preserving techniques, and the German-Austrian-Swiss network FertiPROTECKT (www.fertiprotekt.com), which is a network of approximately 125 centres (as of 2019) that offer fertility preservation for cancer and non-cancer patients.

5.2.3 The Experience of Oocyte Cryopreservation in the United States

Following a thorough review of literature and assessment of short-term maternal and neonatal outcomes, the ASRM practice committee lifted the experimental label on planned oocyte cryopreservation in 2012. Following further research on the efficacy, which was reassuring, the Association of Reproductive Managers ethics committee approved planned oocyte cryopreservation as ethically permissible. There have been significant arguments 'for' and 'against' planned oocyte freezing. Increasing reproductive options, enhancing women's autonomy, a procedure offering 'beneficence' and promoting social justice were debated for promoting planned oocyte cryopreservation. The lack of long-term safety aspects, the cost effectiveness, the possibility of offering a false sense of security, and negative influence on societal aspects were considered drawbacks of this procedure.

A retrospective observational cohort study conducted at a single large university-affiliated centre in the United States between 2006 and 2020 observed that only 7.4% of patients returned to use their oocytes and the cumulative live birth rate per patient who initiated the thawing-warming cycle was 32.4%. None of the women aged 40 or over had a successful outcome with autologous cryopreserved oocytes (Leung et al, 2021).

A large retrospective study analysis based on SART data using 54,667 oocyte cryopreservation cycles and 6,413 oocyte thaw cycles between 2012 and 2018 gives an insight on the trend of oocyte cryopreservation cycles in the United States. There was a significant increase in oocyte cryopreservation cycles between 2012 and 2018, from 2,719 to 13,824, with an increase in oocyte thaw treatment cycles from 348 to 1,810. While age at the time of oocyte cryopreservation remains stable, maternal age at the time of oocyte thaw increased from 36.0 (standard deviation 5.6) to 38.5 (5). The average duration of cryopreservation at the time of oocyte thaw was 15.7 months (standard deviation 19.7) to 29.4 (28.10), from 2012 to 2018. The average number of oocytes per retrieval, the average number of oocytes per thawed cycle, and the average number of embryos available for transfer decreased with an increase in female age at the time of oocyte cryopreservation. The number of oocytes per live birth increased from 41.4 (women <35) to 122.4 (>42 years of age). One drawback of this study was that most women in this study underwent oocyte cryopreservation as part of infertility treatment rather than for family planning purposes.

Another retrospective cohort study to evaluate outcomes of planned oocyte cryopreservation was conducted using data between 2005 and 2009 (Blakemore et al, 2021). This study had a total of 231 patients (280 cycles) with a mean age of 38.2 years (range 23–45) at the time of the first oocyte retrieval. It concluded that the utilisation rate following planned oocyte cryopreservation was 38.1%, and the 'no-use' rate was 58.9%, which was similar across different age groups. The no-use rate was considered a surprising finding, which was consistent across the ages, arguing against the recommendation of oocyte cryopreservation at younger ages. A recent study suggested that treatment cycles using autologous, previously cryopreserved oocytes are in the ranges of 3.1–9.3%, projecting the cost effectiveness to USD 600K–1 million.

A further retrospective study conducted at a single centre evaluated 1,283 vitrified oocytes that were subsequently warmed for 128 autologous IVF treatment cycles between January 2009 and April 2012 (Doyle et al, 2015). A total of 2,994 vitrified blastocysts were warmed for transfer. The percentages of live-born children per warmed blastocyst, according to patient age at the time of oocyte retrieval and blastocyst cryopreservation, ranged from 35.9% for women aged <30 years to 13.3% for women aged 43 to 44 years. The authors recommend cryopreserving 15–20 metaphase II oocytes for women aged <38 years (giving them roughly 70–80% chance of at least one live birth) and 25–30 metaphase II oocytes for women aged 38–40 years (giving them roughly 65–75% chance of at least one live birth).

5.2.4 The Experience of Oocyte Cryopreservation in Australia

The Australasian CREI Consensus Expert Panel on Trial Evidence group (ANZSREI ACCEPT) met in 2017 and 2018 to identify clinical aspects relating to care for elective oocyte cryopreservation. Oocyte cryopreservation for medical and non-medical reasons is available in Australia. The demand for this technique is increasing and fuelled by the increasing number of Australian women delaying childbearing, resulting in a rise in the median age of mothers and a decline in Australia's total fertility rate. The Australian and New Zealand Assisted Reproduction Database reports that a growing number of Australian women are opting for oocyte cryopreservation. The ANZSREI ACCEPT group recommends that the term 'social egg freezing' be replaced by 'elective' or 'planned egg freezing'.

5.2.5 The Experience of Oocyte Cryopreservation in the Middle East and North Africa Region

Despite a rise in population, the fertility rates have decreased from 7 children per woman in 1960 to less than 3 in 2020. As per data from the International Labour Organization, the overall female workforce participation in the Middle East and North Africa (MENA) region is on the rise. From 1990 to 2019, the female workforce ratio increased 24% in the United Arab Emirates, 7% in Saudi Arabia, and 15% in Oman, while a 3% decrease was noted in Egypt. Along with other trends seen related to an increase in oocyte cryopreservation technique, reasons specific to the MENA region include a shift of infertility seen as taboo to an acceptable option, an increase in literacy rates, and the use of contraception and changes in cultural norms. In the MENA region, the majority of infertility treatments are concentrated around the United Arab Emirates, Saudi Arabia, and Egypt.

With the exception of Iran and Lebanon (2017 data), the majority of IVF labs in the MENA region did not allow routine freezing of oocytes. This was in view of the religious laws prohibiting gamete donation. The new IVF law in the United Arab Emirates allows fertility preservation by an unmarried woman to freeze oocytes for five years (which may be extendable on request).

5.2.6 The Experience of Oocyte Cryopreservation in Asia

The majority of Asian countries have joined the Asian Society for Fertility Preservation. Japan, Korea, India, China, and Singapore have established fertility societies. The guidelines vary between these nations based on the individual country's social, religious, and economic aspects.

International professional networks providing data collation and professional exchange include the special interest group 'fertility preservation' of ESHRE and ASRM, the oncofertility consortium (www.oncofertility.northwestern.edu) and the International Society for Fertility Preservation (www.isfp-fertility.org).

5.3 Long-Term Outcomes from Oocyte Freezing

The crucial step and rate-limiting clinical aspect are controlled ovarian stimulation and associated aspects common to the conventional ART treatments. The safety of these techniques has been widely established. The current evidence, per se, does not indicate that oocyte cryopreservation is associated with an increase in adverse maternal or neonatal outcomes. Despite the lack of long-term follow-up studies, the causality of association of any adverse outcome is attributed to the process of IVF in general. Investigation of additional factors to assess cryopreservation protocols and agents, the physical stress on the oocytes frozen, the cellular responses to cryopreservation, and issues relating to freezing and warming processes are warranted.

Alteration in epigenetics of embryos created from cryopreserved oocytes has been investigated in animal models, with varying conclusions. It is debatable whether these changes may be applied to human embryos. Other logistical aspects to be considered include restrictions in the time period for storage (e.g., there is a 10-year limit on storing oocytes for non-medical reasons), the reduced cost effectiveness and increase in personal regret following failure to use the oocytes, and the risk of losing frozen oocytes due to a failure in the freezing mechanism.

5.3.1 Outcomes for Women Undergoing Controlled Ovarian Stimulation

The risks associated with oocyte cryopreservation are similar to those undergoing conventional IVF treatments. Fortunately, with advancements in clinical medicine and laboratory techniques, the risks are very low. Women should be aware of risks associated with anaesthesia and oocyte retrieval like pelvic infection, damage to pelvic organs, blood loss, and ovarian torsion. The most serious complication following controlled ovarian stimulation is the risk of ovarian hyperstimulation syndrome. However, with increasing use of antagonist-based controlled ovarian stimulation regimes with an agonist trigger for final oocyte maturation, the risk is low. Women should also be aware of the financial implications of the need for multiple attempts at controlled ovarian stimulation and frozen embryo transfers. Several demographic and treatment factors influence maternal and neonatal outcomes. The demographic factors include maternal age and pre-treatment body mass index (BMI), race and ethnicity, smoking status, number of oocytes, the number and stage of the embryos transferred, and the type of protocols used for the frozen embryo transferred.

5.3.2 Maternal Outcomes Following Oocyte Cryopreservation

It is well known and well documented that the maternal and neonatal outcomes following IVF treatment are related to advanced maternal age, multiple-order pregnancy (following multiple embryo transfer), and intrinsic biological factors associated with the underlying infertility diagnosis. The majority of women undergoing oocyte cryopreservation are of advanced age. Both maternal and neonatal risks following oocyte cryopreservation may be higher as women return for treatment at a more advanced age. The degree of attrition from oocyte to embryo increases with age, and each resulting embryo has a lower chance of implantation. The implanted embryo also has a higher chance of miscarriage based on the female age at the time of cryopreservation. The major limiting factor for the lack of high-quality data following oocyte cryopreservation treatment is the underutilisation of frozen oocytes.

Recent evidence suggests that the presence or absence of a corpus luteum could be responsible for the suboptimal maternal and neonatal outcomes after a frozen embryo transfer. As women invariably undergo a frozen embryo transfer to achieve a pregnancy following oocyte cryopreservation, we conducted a systematic review and meta-analysis of observational cohort studies (*Data Sources: PubMed, Cochrane registry, Embase, Scopus, and Web of Science were searched through Jan 10, 2022; Search Strategy: (natural OR stimulated OR hormone OR modified OR artificial) AND (frozen OR thawed OR vitrified OR warmed OR cryopreserved) AND embryo AND transfer*) to investigate the mean differences in endometrial thickness, maternal and neonatal outcomes in a natural cycle (NC) compared to a hormone replacement therapy (HRT) frozen embryo transfer (FET) (Raff et al, 2022). 39 observational cohort studies with 49,913 women who underwent HRT-FET and 50,425 women who underwent a NC-FET met the inclusion criteria in our study. Pooled data suggested that the endometrial thickness in women undergoing HRT was significantly lower than those undergoing NC-FET; the mean difference [confidence interval] was –0.4 [–0.5; –0.3]. In view of significant heterogeneity between studies and to evaluate potential confounding, we performed a subgroup analysis based on maternal age and BMI. There was no significant difference in the mean maternal age, –0.2 yr [–0.5; 0.1], or BMI, 0.2 kg/m^2 [0.0; 0.4], between the HRT and NC-FET groups, increasing the validity of our study findings.

In our systematic review, the odds ratio (95% confidence interval) for the combined analysis for (a) abruptio placenta, (b) placenta previa, (c) Caesarean section rates, (d) ectopic pregnancy rates, (e) gestational diabetes mellitus, (f) hypertensive disorder of pregnancy and the risks of (g) postpartum haemorrhage, (h) preterm delivery <32 weeks and (i) preterm delivery <37 weeks of gestation are shown in Table 5.2.

Table 5.2   Maternal outcomes following frozen embryo transfers in a HRT-FET compared to a Natural Cycle FET.

Outcomes	Heterogeneity – I^2 % (p value)	OR (95% confidence interval)
Abruptio placenta	0 (0.78)	1.6 (1.0;2.5)
Placenta previa	31 (0.15)	1.1 (0.9;1.4)
Caesarean section rates	72 (<0.01)	1.5 (1.4;1.6)
Ectopic pregnancy	55 (<0.01)	1.4 (1.1;1.8)
Gestational diabetes	88 (<0.01)	1.0 (0.8;1.2)
Hypertensive disorder of pregnancy	78 (<0.01)	1.9 (1.6;2.2)
Postpartum haemorrhage	49 (0.08)	2.6 (1.9;3.4)
Preterm delivery <32 weeks	57 (0.02)	1.5 (1.1;2.0)
Preterm delivery <37 weeks	49 (0.01)	1.2 (1.1;1.4)

5.3.3 Neonatal Outcomes Following Oocyte Cryopreservation

Oocyte cryopreservation freezing and protocols remain largely safe. Reproductive biologists should be aware of the role of cryoprotectants in preventing cryo-injuries, the factors affecting cellular response to cryopreservation, and the potential problems arising from cryopreserving and warming mature human oocytes. There is evidence based on animal studies to associate the relation of freezing protocols with DNA methylation, histone modifications, global transcriptional differences, and specific gene differences. However, this was not confirmed in studies using cryopreserved human oocytes. There are no good-quality long-term follow-up studies in children born after oocyte cryopreservation.

Outcomes from large databases of donor oocyte banks suggest no additional concerns explicitly related to oocyte cryopreservation. A large retrospective cohort study from Denmark suggested an increased risk of childhood cancer for those born after FET compared with fertile women (44.4 vs. 17.5 per 100,000 person-years, respectively: hazard ratio, 2.43). An increase in imprinting disorders is also reported following FETs (Hargreave et al, 2019).

Emerging evidence suggests that neonatal outcomes may be related to the type of endometrial preparation protocols, specifically in the presence (a natural or modified NC) or absence of a corpus luteum (artificial cycle using HRT). The odds ratio/mean differences (where applicable) (95% confidence interval) for the combined analysis for (a) birth weight >4000 gm, (b) birth weight <2500 gm, (c) large for gestational age, (d) small for gestational age, (e) neonatal mortality, (f) stillbirth, and (g) the differences (standard deviation) for mean gestational age and (h) mean birth weight are shown in Table 5.3.

Our systematic review and meta-analysis stratified outcomes based on singleton pregnancy and twin pregnancies/unspecified outcomes (Raff et al, 2022). Further subgroup analysis was performed using

Table 5.3 Neonatal outcomes following frozen embryo transfers in a HRT-FET compared to a Natural Cycle FET.

Outcomes	Heterogeneity – I^2 % (p value)	OR (95% confidence interval)
Birth weight >4000 gm	58 (<0.01)	1.2 (1.1;1.4)
Birth weight <2500 gm	88 (<0.01)	1.2 (1.0;1.4)
Large for gestational age	88 (<0.01)	1.2 (1.0;1.4)
Small for gestational age	77 (<0.01)	1.1 (1.0;1.3)
Neonatal mortality rate	0 (0.92)	1.2 (0.4;3.8)
Stillbirth rate	47 (0.06)	1.3 (0.7;2.2)
	Heterogeneity – I^2 % (p value)	Mean Difference (95% confidence interval)
Mean gestational age	89 (<0.01)	0 (–0.01;0.2)
Mean birth weight	94 (<0.01)	59 (29.8;88.1)

maternal age and BMI. However, we did not have specific data for FET following oocyte cryopreservation. Women who had treatment in the HRT-FET group consistently showed suboptimal outcomes. We can postulate that HRT may have a role in increasing the suboptimal maternal and neonatal outcomes. Therefore, when analysing the long-term maternal and neonatal outcomes, one should consider the FET treatment protocol.

5.4 Societal Implications

Oocyte cryopreservation raises several social and psychological aspects for women. One criticism of the oocyte cryopreservation technique is that a low number of women return to use their cryopreserved oocytes. The reason for this decline is attributed to natural conception or a decision not to pursue pregnancy. While there are studies suggesting that up to 88% of women are happy with the decision to undergo oocyte cryopreservation and feel control over their reproductive planning, there are other studies that suggest women regret their decision due to a lack of adequacy of information and emotional support, and factors relating to financial constraints. As women undergoing oocyte cryopreservation are emotionally vulnerable, financial and health psychology counselling should be an integral part of the process. Health professionals should help women take an evidence-based decision after getting informed consent for the process.

5.5 Conclusion

Oocyte cryopreservation is considered a preventive intervention for a wide range of medical and non-medical indications. Clearly, the oocyte cryopreservation technique raises significant debates about cultural, ethical, religious, and economic aspects. While there will be significant challenges for political and healthcare policymakers, with growing demand this technique will remain an essential discipline for reproductive biologists, endocrinologists, and the wider medical fraternity of oncologists and health psychologists. Medical professionals should engage in Continuing Medical Education and continue collecting and reporting data nationally and internationally to associate the short- and long-term implications and outcomes of oocyte cryopreservation.

Childlessness is associated with social stigma in many cultures. With the trend of a global decline in population, infertility is not far from being classified as a 'killer disease of the human race', maybe over the next century. Therefore, for the carefully selected patient and with counselling and patient education, oocyte cryopreservation may become a standard 'effective' treatment option within the field of reproductive medicine in the near future.

References

Blakemore JK, Grifo JA, DeVore SM, Hodes-Wertz B, Berkeley AS. Planned oocyte cryopreservation-10-15-year follow-up: return rates and cycle outcomes. Fertil Steril. 2021 Jun;115(6):1511–20.

Cobo A, García-Velasco JA, Remohí J, Pellicer A. Oocyte vitrification for fertility preservation for both medical and nonmedical reasons. Fertil Steril. 2021 May;115(5):1091–101.

Doyle JO, Richter KS, Lim J, Stillman RJ, Graham JR, Tucker MJ. Successful elective and medically indicated oocyte vitrification and warming for autologous in vitro fertilization, with predicted birth probabilities for fertility preservation according to number of cryopreserved oocytes and age at retrieval. Fertil Steril. 2016 Feb;105(2):459–66.e2.

Hargreave M, Jensen A, Hansen MK, Dehlendorff C, Winther JF, Schmiegelow K, Kjær SK. Association between fertility treatment and cancer risk in children. JAMA. 2019 Dec 10;322(22):2203–10.

Johnston M, Richings NM, Leung A, Sakkas D, Catt S. A major increase in oocyte cryopreservation cycles in the USA, Australia and New Zealand since 2010 is highlighted by younger women but a need for standardized data collection. Hum Reprod. 2021 Feb 18;36(3):624–35.

Kakkar P, Geary J, Stockburger T, Kaffel A, Kopeika J, El-Toukhy T. Outcomes of social egg freezing: a cohort study and a comprehensive literature review. J Clin Med. 2023 Jun 21;12(13):4182.

Leung AQ, Baker K, Vaughan D, Shah JS, Korkidakis A, Ryley DA, Sakkas D, Toth TL. Clinical outcomes and utilization from over a decade of planned oocyte cryopreservation. Reprod Biomed Online. 2021 Oct;43(4):671–9.

Raff M, Jacobs EA, Summers KM, Ten Eyck P, Sparks AE, Van Voorhis BJ, Eapen A. Early pregnancy outcomes in hormone replacement therapy and natural cycle frozen embryo transfer following in vitro fertilization treatment: A systematic review and meta-analysis. Fertil Steril. 2022 Apr;118(4):e154.

Tozzo P, Fassina A, Nespeca P, Spigarolo G, Caenazzo L. Understanding social oocyte freezing in Italy: a scoping survey on university female students' awareness and attitudes. Life Sci Soc Policy. 2019 May 3;15(1):3.

Wennberg AL, Schildauer K, Brännström M. Elective oocyte freezing for nonmedical reasons: A 6-year report on utilization and in vitro fertilization results from a Swedish center. Acta Obstet Gynecol Scand. 2019 Nov;98(11):1429–34.

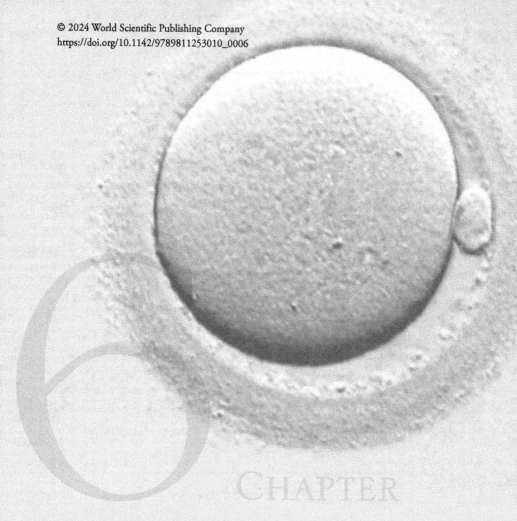

CHAPTER 6

Social Egg Freezing from a UK Perspective:
Can it Help Keep us Warm in the Coming 'Demographic Winter'?

Gillian Lockwood

6.1 Introduction

When, in 2002, my clinic announced the birth of the UK's first baby born following cryopreservation and thawing of a woman's own oocytes for use in an intra-cytoplasmic sperm injection (ICSI)-*in vitro* fertilisation (IVF) cycle, there was a furore in the popular media and some disquiet within the scientific and regulatory establishment (Lockwood, 2002). A bishop announced that I was a 'dangerous woman' trying to 'destroy the family', and he speculated that there would be 'thousands' of 'elderly' single women having babies using their frozen eggs. At the time this seemed somewhat resonant of the anxiety expressed when the oral contraceptive pill was first introduced and finally provided safe and reliable control over their fertility to young women who had previously faced the anxiety of unwanted pregnancy or the stigma and penury of single motherhood. Twenty years on, it is difficult to imagine the mindset that saw the development of egg freezing as anything other than exciting and liberating.

Historically, there have been four major areas in fertility treatment, in which oocyte cryopreservation is appropriate and the first three seem non-controversial. Egg freezing for young single women about to undergo chemotherapy, radiotherapy or surgery for malignancy offers them a chance of a future genetic pregnancy and provides parity with what has been offered to young men who have been able to freeze sperm for decades. Multiple gynaecological conditions such as severe endometriosis, polycystic ovarian syndrome with recurrent cysts and dermoid cysts can severely hamper reproductive options even if they do not represent actual malignancy. A strong female family history of early menopause, especially if corroborated by a poor ovarian reserve test, can also be justification for 'medical' rather than 'social' egg freezing. Egg freezing for women intending to transition to identifying as male but who want to retain some genetic parental potential is another quasi medical justification for egg freezing.

Egg freezing may also offer a prospect of parenthood to couples who have ethical or religious objections to the creation and discarding or cryopreservation of supernumerary embryos. The point at which a human life begins has been variously set from the moment of fertilisation, through to implantation, primitive streak development, quickening, viability, birth or even in some societies after birth, where infanticide was seen as acceptable. During the period when Italian law required all embryos created in a fresh cycle to be transferred and embryo cryopreservation was not permitted, there was intense pressure to improve the pregnancy rates from the surplus eggs that could neither be fertilised, transferred or frozen as embryos. These frozen-thawed oocytes made a valuable contribution to the cumulative pregnancy rate and demonstrated that stopping the biological clock for older would-be mothers could give them the opportunity of healthy pregnancies at a relatively advanced age.

Poor ovarian reserve associated with a low response to ovarian stimulation and the production of few oocytes, often of poor quality, is an increasingly common diagnosis in fertility clinics. Genetic testing of retrieved oocytes prior to and after fertilisation has improved the outcome in terms of viable pregnancy per embryo transfer, but a common outcome is that there are no euploid (chromosomally normal) embryos available for transfer. Hence, for many women the chosen route to motherhood lies with donor eggs. Cryopreservation by vitrification of donor eggs allows for quarantine and matching on whatever basis the local legislation requires. In the UK anonymity for gamete (egg and sperm) donors was abandoned in 2005 and children born as a result of gamete or embryo donation have a legal right to identifying information about their donor upon reaching the age of 18. A right that can obviously only be asserted if their legal parent or parents have shared their 'donor' origins with them: there is no legal compulsion to identify parentage on a birth registration document. The globalisation of the frozen gamete market has added the complication that even though the donor may have recorded accurately their true biographical details, family medical history, passport number and current address in order to fulfil UK requirements for donor identifiability in the future, 18 years later it might prove difficult for a donor-conceived person to find their genetic parent, even if they know to look. The growth in the use of direct-to-consumer genetic tests may result in many individuals discovering information about their genetic origins that was not shared with them, but also the prospect of finding genetic siblings or half-siblings whose existence and contact they may welcome.

Much of the furore concerning frozen eggs relates to 'social' egg freezing, a somewhat derogatory term that I believe should be resisted not least because of the associations with social media but because it denigrates the motives of women who recognise that it may represent their only chance of genetic motherhood. The circumstances in which women choose to freeze eggs often reflect their social situation, in which they have either failed to find a partner who wishes to parent with them or a long-term relationship that they assumed was heading towards parenthood has failed, often because of commitment issues but sometimes due to illness, caring responsibilities or employment demands. It is biologically unfair and socially unfortunate that at the age of 38 (the modal age at which UK women seek 'social' egg freezing), she has two years realistically to achieve a healthy pregnancy whereas her similarly aged male partner has two decades. Studies of graduate couples have shown a similar mismatch between the age at which women feel they would like a first baby (35) and expect to have had their last (40+) and that of their male partners, who will usually be the same age as they met at college, who nevertheless resolutely add at least 5 years to these age targets and also still express a somewhat unrealistic desire to have 'two or three' children (Svanberg et al, 2006).

6.2 Possible Explanations for 'The Baby Shortage' in the UK

To understand why egg freezing may come to be seen as an obvious technological response to a significant biological, social and economic problem, the considerable shifts in socio-economic and reproductive behaviour during the last few decades need to be appreciated. Increasing numbers of people are either postponing parenthood, choosing not to embark on it at all or failing to achieve it due to a complex combination of reasons that include (especially for young women) extended educational and career aspirations, later marriage, more frequent marital and relationship breakdown and changing attitudes to material assets such that personal fulfilment may be attainable by routes other than parenthood. There are perceived barriers to achieving an idealised image of parenthood that involves prerequisite goals in housing, lifestyle and career. Social media and the anonymity of online forums have changed the way we see and talk about motherhood. Financial constraints and especially the high cost of childcare have forced many couples to resign themselves to having an 'only lonely' child or (usually) the mother gives up her job to provide the necessary early-years childcare before returning to (probably) a part-time and/or lower paid job. Since an average UK adult spends 3+ hours a day online (not in gainful employment such as working from home) but on social media, the search for positivity about having a child inevitably results in a flood of glowing images of beautiful babies cradled by equally beautiful mothers in filtered Instagram and TikTok nirvanas that seem, to many, unachievable (Keim, 2011). These edited images have been shown to add unnecessary pressure for would-be mothers and lead to higher rates of depression and anxiety for those who view them. These two polarised views of parenthood may in some way account for the fact that 50% of all British women aged 30 are now child-free and 19% will still not have had a child by the age of 45. Experts in digital ethics are aware of the impact of social media on our real-life decisions. Our social decisions are influenced by the opinions of friends and family and the revelations of celebrities and influencers, but the algorithms that drive social media and that constantly reinforce the images we spend most time looking at change our perceptions of what we want and what we can achieve.

Despite educational campaigns to highlight the risks associated with delaying having babies, the public are more influenced by media images of celebrities that imply that late motherhood is achievable if a healthy lifestyle is pursued: their use of donor eggs is rarely mentioned. That the very real extensions in lifespan that have been achieved in the last 50 years cannot be readily translated into equivalent extensions in reproductive lifespan is neither well understood nor accepted by a society that claims that '40 is the new 30!'. The reproductive lifespan inequality between men and women has long been regarded as regrettable but inevitable, but perhaps it need not be. With women's longer and healthier lifespan, using their own frozen eggs to achieve a pregnancy at a time of their choosing would seem to be no more 'unnatural and undesirable' than making a woman go through an ICSI cycle because her partner has severe male factor infertility. Women who seek 'social' egg freezing are not doing so because they have other life goals and will get around to motherhood when the time is right, but mainly because they have a highly conventional view of parenthood and want to have the opportunity to become a mother in a supportive, long-term relationship (Baldwin, 2015).

6.3 Relationship Problems: Spoiled for Choice?

Some opponents of 'social' egg freezing have claimed that women who choose to freeze their eggs because they have not yet found a suitable co-parent may become too choosy about selecting a possible future partner if they feel immune from the ticking of their biological clock. Apparently 50% of current relationships are started online via dating apps where an algorithm will help you find 'The One', so I describe this anxiety as the 'Sunday Country Pub Lunch Paradox'. This typically English scenario is that a group of friends set off on a sunny Sunday morning to have lunch at an archetypal English country pub. They soon see a suitable hostelry, but it is still quite early and so they drive on confidently expecting something even nicer. The next pub looks perfect, but a small sign on the gate says 'private party today' and so, disappointed, they drive on. Twenty minutes later a beautiful pub comes into view, but the carpark is full to overflowing and it is clear that, even if they can get a table, food will be many hours away. The next pub looks miserable and bar snacks is all they are offered. They eventually settle for sandwiches at a petrol station... I hesitate to suggest that this is analogous to women who have frozen their eggs returning eventually to use them with donor sperm, but the current data suggests that usage rates for 'socially' frozen eggs are quite low. It is reassuring that studies which have looked at usage rates have found that the majority of women who freeze their eggs for either 'social' or gonadotoxic reasons will achieve a pregnancy but, for the overwhelming majority, these will be spontaneous pregnancies or pregnancies achieved with more conventional fertility treatment (De Vos, 2018; Balkenende et al, 2018; Blakemore et al, 2021).

It is increasingly clear that housing status has a huge role to play in determining individuals' reproductive plans. Notwithstanding a legal obligation on UK Councils to provide suitable accommodation for families with children, the shortage of social housing means that even families who are dependent on welfare benefits struggle to be offered suitable accommodation, and young childless couples and individuals are at the mercy of the private rental sector. Young couples, even if they are both in paid employment, may fail to find rented accommodation near to where they work, and many have the aspiration to own their own home (albeit with a large mortgage) with some outside space or garden before starting a family. Rent currently accounts for 30–40% of take-home pay in many regions and that leaves little income to save for a deposit for a property purchase. For fortunate aspiring young homeowners, the 'Bank of Mum and Dad' may be able to help, and in 2021 49% of first-time buyers were aided by parents or family with an average of £58,000 per supported purchase. The average house in the UK currently costs around nine times average (pre-tax) earnings although there are regions where housing is much less expensive, but wages there are often lower too. It is small comfort to know that the ratio has not been this bad for would-be homeowners since the latter half of the 19th century. During the 1950s to 1970s the ratio was more manageable at 4–5 times average earnings and the house price rises since are where the parental equity has been accrued. Half of all babies may well be made by 'accident' rather than design, but for conscientious couples who want a secure home to bring up their baby, housing costs remain a significant block to starting a family and militate against 'happy accidents'.

6.4 The Role of Longer, Higher and Further Education

Globally, it is recognised that educating girls is the most effective way to reduce early marriage, improve maternal and childhood morbidity and mortality, increase economic participation, and reduce family size. In the UK, the proportion of the female population who had no qualifications at the end of compulsory schooling (generally at age 16) decreased from 64% of women born in 1940–1949 to 18% of women born in 1960–1968 (HESA, 2020). For the same cohorts, the proportion of women who earned an academic degree or similar higher-level qualification rose from 9% to 20%. In countries such as the UK, since the late 1990s there has been a policy of encouraging at least 50% of school-leavers to go on to university and girls are more likely both to go to university and to complete their degrees. However, this higher education, which was free when only 10% of school leavers went to university, now is generally paid for by the students themselves by way of student loans, with further loans required for maintenance costs. Maintenance support is dependent on parental household income, with students from the poorest households being exempt, but the average student will graduate with a debt of £45,000. Student loans become repayable once the graduate is earning just 30% above the minimum wage and for those who never attain that threshold the debt will eventually be written off after 30 years. Student loan repayments therefore provide another barrier to financial independence and access to the housing market that impacts most heavily on young women who may be caught in a trap where only low status employment will keep them below the student loan repayment threshold. Mortgage providers should not include student loan debt in decisions about the provision of mortgages for house or flat purchase, but the mere existence of the debt is recognised to have a negative impact on young people's aspirations for their future and their potential family.

The COVID-19 pandemic halved the number of UK marriages in 2021 compared to the previous year but in the 30 years previously between 1989–2019 there had already been a 61% decrease (ONS, 2021). The number of cohabiting couple families continued to grow faster than married couples and lone-parent families, with an increase of 25.8% over the decade 2008 to 2018. Married or civil partner couple families remain the most common type of family in which dependent children live (63.5%) followed by 21.1% in lone-parent families and 15.3% in cohabiting couple families. Another factor is the significant increase in the number of young adults aged 20–34 years living with their parents which now, post COVID, exceeds 25%. There has been a gradual long-term decline in both the number of marriages and marriage rates since the early 1970s. Since 1972 the number of opposite-sex marriages has decreased by 46.7% while marriage rates have fallen by 76.1% for men and 70.7% for women.

Before the pandemic, the average age at marriage was continuing the overall rise recorded since the 1970s, 40 years of age for men and 37 years for women. In terms of the impact of these data on predictable birth rates, it must be recognised that many marriages at older ages may reflect a second marriage after divorce or cohabiting relationship and the over 65s are also marrying at increasing ages. The pandemic also impacted divorce rates with a 10% increase to the highest number seen since 2013. For couples who married in the 1960s, 23% had divorced by their 25th anniversary whereas for more recently married couples only just under half reached their 25th anniversary. The number of marriages ending before their 10th anniversary, the most usual window for parenthood, also increased to 25% for couples marrying in 1995.

6.5 Restructuring the Family

Current family structures in the UK have a significant impact on decisions about the possibility and timing of pregnancy and hence on the appeal of egg freezing. Before the invention of the bicycle permitted ordinary people in small towns and villages to widen their social horizons, couples were usually introduced by family or local friends and settled down to live near to where they were born. Households were often multi-generational with young couples and their babies living under the parental roof and often sharing the hearth with a grandparent. Characteristically the gap between the generations was 20–25 years, so a grandmother would be at most 45–50 when her first grandchild appeared. She would be available to support the new mother and often provide essential free childcare to allow the mother to return to local and probably part-time work. As single generational living became the norm and people were increasingly likely to move away from where they were born to find work and independent accommodation, this vital support network was strained and often broken. The age of first birth also impacts on vertical family structure as a 35-year or even 40-year gap between mother and child is increasingly the norm and women having 'late' babies may find that they are part of the 'sandwich' generation with nurturing responsibility not only for young children whilst in their 50s and teenagers in their 60s, but also caring responsibilities for elderly and possibly frail parents of 80 and beyond. Too often this will be combined with the necessity of a full-time job that may require a daily commute.

One of the most beautiful relationships within families is that between grandparent and grandchild. Grandparents historically had the time, skills and unconditional love to provide care and guidance for grandchildren as part of their extended family. But what baby or toddler could be safely left with a grandmother who is over 80 years old and possibly in need of support and supervision herself? Egg freezing may exacerbate this widening gap between the generations, and we know that babies of older mothers are likely to be 'only' children as having a second child is either biologically or financially unlikely. For some of today's parents of young adults, especially if they come from the 'Boomer' (post-World War 2 baby boom) generation blessed with affordable house prices and generous occupational pensions, becoming a grandparent may be seen as an essential social rite of passage to which they actively aspire. A significant proportion of egg freezing cycles are funded by the parents of single thirty-something daughters. Indeed the 'Bank of would-be grandma and grandad' probably funds many more egg freezing cycles than the highly publicised initiatives of companies such as Facebook and Google which offer egg freezing to their female employees as a perk like gym membership or private health care.

6.6 The Development of Egg Freezing in the UK

Egg freezing cycles are one of the fastest growing treatments in the UK with 11 times more in 2021 (4,215) than in 2011 (373). But this still only represents 4% of fertility treatments, and the data does not distinguish between the reason (medical or 'social') and the source of funding (government, private or employer funded) (HFEA, 2021). Big tech companies were amongst the first to include egg freezing as a work benefit, and there was an initial backlash against this somewhat dystopian vision of encouraging valuable female employees to defer having babies in the interests of their careers and the company's profits. An overwhelming body of research evidence confirms that it is the absence of a partner and/or the financial constraints of housing and childcare costs that prevent young women from having babies in their late 20s and early 30s and not an irresistible career imperative (Inhorn, 2023). I was genuinely appalled to be told by a delegate of a merchant bank considering offering egg freezing as a 'perk' to their female employees who had been in post for more than five years that, 'Management prefers experienced young women to recent graduates or peri-menopausal crones'. My suggestion that perhaps they should consider subsidised workplace nurseries and more flexible working patterns for these valuable employees was met with derision. It is highly significant that the employees most likely to be offered the 'perk' of egg freezing or to avail themselves of it with personal funding are not representative of the female workforce in general.

6.7 The 'Demographic Winter' is Coming

The interaction between economics and fertility is subtle but significant. It is well recognised that in developed countries poorer women tend to have higher fertility rates and this is mistakenly taken as evidence that poverty somehow promotes high fertility. This argument was compounded by the apparent bias in welfare programmes that historically seemed to reward feckless fecundity and conspire to trap large families in a dependency culture where payments received in response to high numbers of children would inevitably exceed what their parents could earn as part of the labour force. In an attempt to thwart this behaviour, the UK capped the number of children whose families were eligible for many welfare benefits at two children per household. Another way of interpreting the association between poverty and fecundity is that women who have large families or have children earlier tend to end up poorer. The 'fertility penalty', that is the loss in lifetime earnings as a result of time out of the labour market, is actually higher for low-skilled women than for mid-skilled or professional women. This is because lower-skilled women will be away

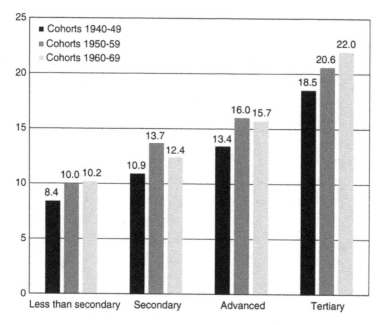

Figure 6.1   Childlessness by birth cohort (in %) and highest level of education for British women aged 40–49 born 1940–1969. Source: General Household Survey.

from work longer (because of extra pregnancies and unaffordable childcare) and may need to accept very low paid work to get the shorter or more flexible hours they need to return to work at all. Using educational attainment as a surrogate marker for socio-economic status (see Figure 6.1), it is clear that for women, possession of a degree doubles the chance of childlessness.

The lower fertility rates of women from higher sectors of the socio-economic spectrum and their lower 'fertility penalties' are perceived as the result of undertaking higher education and training for careers that offer better prospects, such as generous maternity leave and pay, flexible working and maintenance of a position on the career ladder. Within many developed countries, and notably within the UK, the accelerating trend for delaying parenthood is overlaid by a marked difference between fertility rates in differing socio-economic groups within the same society. Analysis of data derived from the British Birth Cohort Study (BCS70) which followed babies born in one week in April 1970 looked at fertility outcomes. It was found that 60% of men and 46% of women born in 1970 were childless at age 30, but far higher proportions of degree-educated man and women were childless at age 30 (80% of graduate men and 69% of graduate women) (Berrington and Pattaro, 2014). Adults from this cohort who reported childlessness at 30 were re-surveyed at age 42 and 73% of the men and 80% of the women responded. Eventually, by the age of 42, 75% of men and 80% of women will have had at least one child. What is quite clear from the data, however, is that the chance of childlessness for women who have received a tertiary level education is far higher than for women without qualifications. It is equally significant that highly educated males showed the greatest tendency to postpone parenthood and the predicted rate of childlessness for males in this group is 27% (Elliot and Shepherd, 2006). The increasing delay at entry to fatherhood and male childlessness are important aspects of the shifting pattern of parenting in Britain today and seem to bear out the oft-repeated lament that educated men are commitment phobic about relationships and having children, at least in having children with a partner who is close in age to them. This may be a partial, if uncomfortable, explanation for the increase in 'social' egg freezing currently being seen.

It would appear then that an increasingly numerically and economically significant group of young adults are moving inexorably towards an ambivalent attitude to parenthood/childlessness which could be described as perpetual postponing. Both women and men, especially if they have received a tertiary-level education and professional training and have good employment prospects, are currently living in a society which is not designed to help them cope with the narrow time-window of opportunity for becoming parents that exists in the decade between realisation of educational, career and economic goals and the onset of the prospect of a small family or involuntary childlessness. These women maintain a strong latent desire for motherhood, but do not or cannot act until it is too late in biological time. The increase in perpetual postponers has led to greater reliance on assisted conception but, as the data shows, even with IVF, success rates for this group of women in terms of live births are poor and the personal and financial costs are high. Progress has been made in IVF success rates with birth rates per embryo transferred at 33% for patients aged 18–34 and 25% for 38–39-year-olds. For older patients, however, the success rates remain bleak with just 16% for 40–42-year-olds and only 6% for 43–50-year-olds achieving a pregnancy using their own fresh eggs (HFEA, 2021). Berrington's studies have investigated how parental aspirations for education, educational ability in childhood and educational attainment in young adulthood impact significantly on the achievement of fertility intentions. Influenced by their parents' socio-economic background and their educational and employment achievements, this can create an ambivalence towards parenthood which easily turns into perpetual postponing. The majority of little girls may play with dolls and dream of having real babies but there is a clear negative educational gradient in the likelihood of achieving the number of intended births by the time that biological time has run out.

Cryopreservation of a woman's own oocytes perhaps then offers a realistic technological fix for what is essentially a biological and sociological problem. Perhaps people will be appalled at the prospect of women using the technology of ovarian stimulation, vitrification and ICSI to achieve healthy live births of their own genetic babies in their forties when society feels that they should have had those babies naturally in their twenties or early thirties. But these women either were not ready or able to have those babies then. Either they were not in a position to start a family because of socially laudable educational or career goals, or because they had not found the right partner who was willing and able to parent a child with them, or they had health issues or caring responsibilities. When a (high-profile) woman in her mid or even late forties does achieve a healthy birth naturally, often after a characteristic sequence of tragic early miscarriages, the joy expressed is genuine and universal. What can then be wrong in using the technology of egg freezing to help other women achieve this too?

Let us consider a thought experiment. Suppose the same DNA- or RNA-based pharmaceutical breakthroughs that facilitated the development of the anti-COVID vaccines, and arguably saved millions of lives during the pandemic, have been tweaked to allow women to wind back their biological clocks by a decade. A single jab could mean that 40 really is the new 30 in terms of reproductive potential. How does removing the expensive, high-tech wizardry which is egg harvesting, cryopreservation by vitrification and ICSI change the moral and ethical environment here? If we could avoid the expense, risks and uncertainty of egg freezing, would society still be so hostile to the concept of women in their 40s being able to become what men in their 40s and older have always been able to become, that is a parent?

The evidence base in favour of the efficacy and safety of oocyte cryopreservation is overwhelming, especially for younger women who characteristically yield good numbers of high-quality oocytes with low levels of stimulation. Survival rates post-thaw, fertilisation rates with ICSI and implantation rates of young cryopreserved oocytes are strictly comparable with those of matched fresh oocytes and the outcome for mothers and babies are equivalent to ICSI with fresh eggs (HFEA, 2021). In her early forties, when many women are finally in a position to start a family, due to the fact that egg quality declines with age, their chance of a natural conception with their own fresh eggs is low. The miscarriage rate for a woman at 45 is 80% and that is for women who can actually get pregnant. Using her own previously frozen eggs the chance of a healthy live birth at 45 is as good as for a 30-year-old. The age of a woman at freeze is far more significant than her age at thaw. Pregnancies for the over-40s are recognised to be more hazardous with an increased risk of complications such as high blood pressure and diabetes, but these risks are actually lower when the women are using their autologous frozen eggs, their own genetic material, rather than donor eggs.

It is often claimed that fertility preservation by means of egg freezing is acceptable for young single cancer patients facing significantly reduced fertility following chemotherapy or radiotherapy but that this argument somehow does not apply to women seeking 'social' egg freezing. Sterility following cancer therapy is highly unpredictable, however it is absolutely certain that a woman's advancing age much beyond 40 will have an inevitable and seriously deleterious impact on her fertility.

If a woman never needs to use her frozen eggs, or chooses not to, because she achieves her desired number of pregnancies or never finds herself in a position to embark on even one, then the unused eggs may be discarded or donated for research. Some women have claimed that egg freezing represents an 'insurance policy' against future age-related sub-fertility: they may pay the insurance 'premium' hoping that they will never need to claim on the policy. Many women have stated that egg freezing offers an opportunity to be proactive, to assert some agency over a biological process that renders them otherwise helpless. This 'insurance policy' may be an inappropriate analogy, as a healthy pregnancy cannot be guaranteed however many of her frozen eggs are available, but this is exactly the same position faced by any couple trying to conceive naturally or with conventional fertility treatment. After all, we encourage all householders to take out fire insurance even though only a tiny minority will ever need to make a claim.

The British Childhood Survey (BCS70) throws an intriguing light on the psychology of parenting intentions (see Table 6.1) (Berrington, 2017). A surprisingly small group of young people have been identified as 'early articulators' who report from a young age that they do not want to be parents. More encounter 'childlessness through circumstance' or 'social infertility' which describes people who do not find a suitable

Table 6.1   Intention to have a child according to highest level of education among 1970 British Cohort Study members who were childless at age 30. Figures are percentages (n = 2,599). Source: Ann Berrington's analysis of BCS70.

	Yes	Don't know	No	Self/partner not able to have children
Men				
Less than secondary	57.2	22.8	16.3	3.7
Secondary	62.6	21.5	13.1	2.8
Advanced	64.1	22.0	11.5	2.4
Tertiary	69.3	19.3	10.2	1.3
Total	63.5	21.2	12.8	2.5
Women				
Less than secondary	58.1	18.9	15.0	8.1
Secondary	63.2	14.3	14.4	8.0
Advanced	66.8	17.1	11.8	4.3
Tertiary	67.6	19.5	9.7	3.1
Total	64.5	17.4	12.4	5.7

partner or whose partner does not want children. Most studies assume a general infertility rate of 5–8%, but many couples who fulfil the medical definition of infertility, but do not have children, reject the label, perhaps because they fear the stigma or worry that little can be done to help them or they cannot afford to access fertility treatment. In the BCS70 study of still childless 30-year-olds, the respondents were asked whether they intended to have children, with the possible answers being 'yes', 'no' or 'don't know'. Although there was a tendency for higher educated people to express an intention to have at least one child, it is striking that the overwhelming majority (57–69%) of both men and women, irrespective of educational attainment, intended to have a child. A further approximately 20% overall replied 'don't know'.

At age 42 they were asked to provide details of their achieved fertility outcomes and it transpires that, for this significant group of postponers, fertility intentions aged 30 were a good predictor of fertility outcomes. Half of both male and female postponers, those who said they intended to have children, went on to have two or more children whereas those who were undecided at 30 were more likely to remain childless or have just one child. Well-educated postponers were more likely to achieve their desired fertility outcomes and we may speculate on whether their higher socio-economic status, better general health or ability to fund fertility treatment impact on this.

Childless respondents at 42 were asked why they had not (yet) had children and the most common reason was that the respondent had not wanted children (cited by 28% of men and 31% of women). Psychology teaches us that rationalisation of a painful situation is often a chosen coping strategy. The second most common reason was that the respondent had never met the right person (23% of men and 19% of women) but this crucially consisted of 34% of graduate women. Only 5% of women admitted that they had wanted children but had not 'got around to it' and just 2% of all the women (3% of graduate women) cited being focussed on their career as the main reason for their childlessness.

There remain two significant psychological issues that must be addressed in any consideration of 'social' egg freezing. In the UK this may best be described by the phrase taken from fairytales 'one day my Prince will come'. It is perhaps only human nature that women believe that they will be able to have a child, if that is their desire, at a time of their choosing. The current data suggests that this is unlikely to be the case for a significant minority. The other consideration is the status of the unused eggs in the freezer. Recent legislative changes in the UK mean that the original 10-year limit (except for exceptional circumstances such as cancer where longer storage had been allowed) for the storage of eggs has been extended till the egg owner is 55. For some women this has provided a welcome respite from the fear that they must either use their eggs, perhaps with donor sperm, or allow them, and their dreams of motherhood, to perish. But for other women, the presence of these tantalising 'what if' potential babies in the freezer is a source of real concern and despair.

Unlike many Western neighbours, the UK's population is not actually falling as net immigration more than compensates for the low birth rate. The UK population has grown year-on-year since 1980 and recently the annual rises have been around 0.3–0.4% (Macrotrends, 2022). For demographers, the ideal substitution index is 2.1. That is the fertility rate, the number of babies born per woman, that allows the population to remain stable. Regular increases in the retirement age maintains the level of the working population even though the jobs that these would-be pensioners are capable of doing are not necessarily what the economy actually needs. The current UK fertility rate of 1.6 represents an average of the births registered to women born outside the UK (28.7% of all births or a total fertility rate of 1.97) and that of UK-born women (total fertility rate 1.57), but it is clearly far below the ideal substitution index. 'Social' egg freezing clearly cannot solve this problem, but for some of the 34% of graduate women who cite their failure to find a partner before biology has made it unlikely they will be able to have children, it may let them feel that they can safely buy a little biological time. The ideal situation is that couples should be presented with the more positive aspects of parenting, and encouraged to have children sooner rather than later. Society should work towards a social framework that is financially and structurally supportive of young families and where the whole society recognises that nurturing the development of children is a vital societal role for our collective future.

References

Baldwin K, Culley L, Hudson N, Mitchell H, Lavery S. Oocyte cryopreservation for social reasons: demographic profile and disposal intentions of UK users. Reprod Biomed Online. 2015 Aug;31(2): 239–45.

Balkenende EM, Dahhan T, van der Veen F, Repping S, Goddijn M. Reproductive outcomes after oocyte banking for fertility preservation. Reprod Biomed Online. 2018 Oct;37(4):425–33.

Berrington A, Pattaro S. Educational differences in fertility desires, intentions and behaviour: A life course perspective. Adv Life Course Res. 2014 Sep;21:10–27.

Berrington A. Childlessness in the UK. In: Kreyenfeld M, Konietzka D, editors. Childlessness in Europe: contexts, causes and consequences. Springer; 2017. p. 64–66.

Blakemore JK, Grifo JA, DeVore SM, Hodes-Wertz B, Berkeley AS. Planned oocyte cryopreservation-10-15-year follow-up: return rates and cycle outcomes. Fertil Steril. 2021 Jun;115(6):1511–20.

De Vos M. Follow-up of elective oocyte cryopreservation for age related reasons. P523 ESHRE Annual meeting 2018.

Elliott J, Shepherd P. Cohort profile: 1970 British Birth Cohort (BCS70). Int J Epidemiol. 2006 Aug;35(4):836–43.

Fertility treatment 2021: preliminary trends and figures report. https://www.hfea.gov.uk/about-us/publications/research-and-data/fertility-treatment-2021-preliminary-trends-and-figures

HESA Higher Education Standards Statistics 2020/2022. https://www.hesa.ac.uk

Inhorn M. Motherhood on ice: the mating gap and why women freeze their eggs. New York University Press; 2023.

Keim S. Social networks and family formation processes. Springer; 2011.

Lockwood G. Politics, ethics and economics: oocyte cryopreservation in the UK. Reprod Biomed Online. 2003 Mar;6(2):151–3.

Macrotrends 2022. https://www.macrotrends.net/countries/GBR/united-kingdom/population

ONS Office of National Statistics. Marriage in England and Wales 2021. https://www.ons.gov.uk/people

Skoog Svanberg A, Lampic C, Karlström PO, Tydén T. Attitudes toward parenthood and awareness of fertility among postgraduate students in Sweden. Gend Med. 2006 Sep;3(3):187–95.

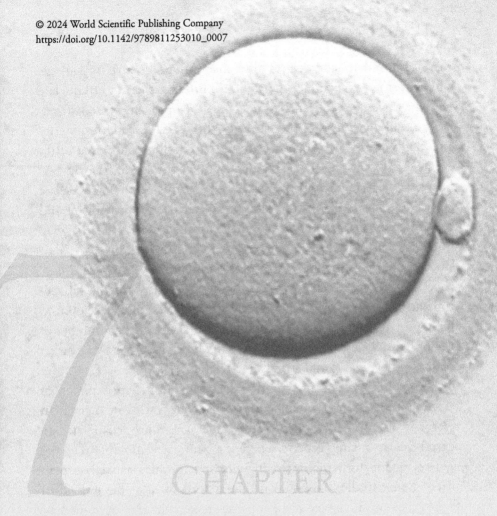

CHAPTER

The Assessment of
Ovarian Reserve Prior to
Oocyte Freezing

Karolina Palinska-Rudzka

There is a fundamental gender difference in reproductive physiology. While most males maintain the ability to produce sperm until the late stages of their lives, all females' oocytes develop during foetal stages. Oocytes, all of which are present at birth, decrease in both quantity and quality over time. There are around 1–2 million oocytes at birth, around 25,000 at the age of 37, and 1,000 at the age of 51, which is the average age of menopause in the UK (Faddy et al, 1992). Most oocytes are enclosed in primordial or so-called 'resting' follicles and can remain at this stage of development for many years. Only a small proportion of primordial follicles are recruited to grow each day. Around 99% of the growing follicles eventually become atretic, while some continue to grow and become responsive to the follicle-stimulating hormone (FSH) and only selected ones may develop into the dominant follicle. There is a progressive decline in the number of primordial follicles throughout a woman's life. The process of ovarian ageing is unavoidable and strictly age-related.

The term ovarian reserve describes the estimated number of oocytes present in a woman's ovaries. A wide variation in ovarian reserve is observed in women of the same age group. It is related to several factors, mainly genetic. There is a clear correlation between the ages of menopause amongst daughters and mothers as well as twin sisters. Some studies have shown that at least 50% of the individual factors accounting for age at menopause are genetic. However, medical and surgical interventions play a significant role, particularly in women with advanced endometriosis and those exposed to chemotherapy and radiotherapy. Smoking cigarettes is another crucial factor associated with earlier menopause and loss of ovarian reserve. Studies have shown a dose- and duration-dependent relationship between smoking and age of menopause. Overall, other lifestyle factors have been estimated to have a small contribution to variation in menopausal age. Age at menarche, parity, regularity of menstrual cycles, use of contraception, breastfeeding, alcohol and coffee consumption, diet, body mass index, and socioeconomic status are all debatable in terms of their effects on menopausal age.

Not only does the quantity but also the quality of oocytes declines with age. Moreover, statistical analyses show that women of an older age are far more likely to have a miscarriage, which is related to the higher incidence of chromosomal abnormalities in embryos. Factors responsible for the declining quality and the higher chances of chromosomal abnormalities in oocytes with age are complex and require further research. Various groups believe that declining quality of cytoplasm in the oocyte and efficiency of DNA damage repairs, as well as instability of mitochondrial DNA and shortening of telomeres, may all play a role. Further evidence comes from clinical experience where older women achieve pregnancy and live birth rates of younger women if they receive donated eggs from a young donor. As a significant variation of oocyte reserve is seen between women, an individual and accurate assessment of the remaining pool of follicles is invaluable in any patient seeking egg freezing. In addition, it facilitates counselling prior to fertility preservation and predicts the number of oocytes retrievable in the ovarian stimulation cycle. Currently, there is a lack of a marker that directly measures the size of a pool of resting follicles. However, this pool is linked to the small cohort of early growing follicles and antral follicles that are more readily measurable (Wallace, 2010). Nevertheless, the perfect ovarian reserve marker has not yet been identified. Ideally, an ovarian reserve test should be highly reproducible and informative of the quantity and quality of oocytes, irrespective of the menstrual cycle phase and the interplay of hormones.

The available ovarian reserve tests can be divided into two groups: biophysical and biochemical. The latter include measurements of an early follicular phase FSH, oestradiol (E2), and Anti-Müllerian hormone (AMH). Biophysical tests involve measuring the antral follicle count (AFC) using transvaginal ultrasound (TV USS). The other indirect measures of the ovarian reserve, e.g., dynamic biochemical tests such as the clomiphene citrate challenge test or TV USS measurements of ovarian volume, are not commonly used in everyday practice. However, emerging evidence favours the use of AMH and AFC, which are valuable for predicting response to ovarian stimulation and are considered the most reliable ovarian reserve markers.

7.1 Follicle-Stimulating Hormone/Oestradiol

FSH is a gonadotropin secreted by the anterior pituitary gland in response to gonadotropin release hormone. It promotes the growth of the ovarian follicles and oestrogen production. The pituitary secretion of FSH varies throughout the cycle and is under E2 and inhibin feedback, so the perfect timing of the blood sample testing is essential. FSH in the early menstrual cycle indicates the tonic level of gonadotrophin stimulation needed to drive the menstrual cycle. As a woman ages and ovarian reserve declines, FSH increases early in the cycle because the pituitary gland must produce more FSH to generate an oestrogen response from the waning ovarian follicle population. E2 is a steroid hormone produced by the aromatisation of androstenedione from theca cells and conversion from estrone into E2. In addition, smaller amounts of precursors are also produced by the adrenal cortex and fat cells (Luesley & Baker, 2004). E2 is involved in the feedback between the growing follicle and the pituitary. High concentrations of E2 early in the menstrual cycle reflect the advanced follicular development and early selection of the dominant follicle. As the ovary ages, day 2–5 E2 is frequently seen to increase transiently before levels drop at menopause.

The basal level of FSH in serum, measured between day two and five of the menstrual cycle, was the most widely used ovarian reserve test in fertility clinics worldwide but recently lost popularity due to its limitations. It is known that increased serum FSH concentrations are observed in the early follicular phase of the menstrual cycle in women with depleted ovarian reserve. Elevated early follicular phase FSH is a highly specific but not particularly sensitive marker of diminished ovarian reserve. In regularly cycling women, the measurement of basal FSH predicts response to ovarian stimulation only at high threshold levels (Broekmans et al, 2006). Furthermore, intra- and inter-cycle variations limit the use of FSH as a marker of ovarian reserve. Those fluctuations in FSH levels become more apparent in older patients. At the same time, the persistent rise in the basal FSH concentration is a late indicator of a decreased follicle pool.

Ideally, basal FSH measurement should be accompanied by serum E2. An elevated E2 level in an early follicular phase can lower FSH, providing false reassurance of 'normal' FSH concentrations and misinterpretation of the ovarian reserve test. Several publications have shown a correlation between elevated levels of an early follicular phase serum E2 and a poor response to ovarian stimulation despite normal basal FSH (Evers et al, 1998).

Basal E2 concentration is a poor predictor of response to ovarian stimulation due to extremely low predictive accuracy and lack of precise threshold levels (Broekmans et al, 2006). Therefore, based on current evidence, early follicular phase E2 cannot be used as a reliable predictor of response to *in vitro* fertilisation (IVF) stimulation or screening test for possible poor responders. In clinical practice, combined measurements of basal FSH and E2 are helpful in the selected group of patients planning egg freezing. However, in a group of patients newly diagnosed with cancer, due to FSH sampling time constraints and low accuracy, other ovarian reserve markers, e.g., AMH or AFC, are considered more suitable.

7.2 Antral Follicle Count

The ovaries of women of reproductive age contain populations of follicles at various stages of development. These are the resting reserve of primordial follicles, recruited early growing follicles (<2 mm), small selectable antral follicles (2–5 mm), larger antral follicles (6–10 mm) and dominant/ovulatory follicles. The number of antral follicles reflects the number of resting follicles in each ovary. Antral follicles, which are >2 mm in diameter, are detectable on USS, but some of them might be already in the initial stages of atresia (Broekmans et al, 2010).

In clinical practice, AFC is the total number of follicles sized between 2–10 mm in both ovaries measured by TV USS. AFC declines steadily till the age of 37 and more rapidly thereafter. AFC was found to be predictive of the number of oocytes collected in response to controlled ovarian stimulation in several trials (Fleming et al, 2015). Typically, measurements occur between days 2 and 5 of the menstrual cycle due to known intracycle variations. However, recent studies suggest that the assessment of AFC at any stage of the menstrual cycle is highly predictive of the number of oocytes retrieved in the IVF cycle (Razafintsalama-Bourdet et al, 2022).

The accuracy of AFC as an ovarian reserve test is impacted by high inter-operator variability and low inter-centre reproducibility. The diversity of methods, including the difference in the ultrasound machine and its settings used and measurements of different groups of follicles (including atretic follicles), impact on the performance of AFC as a diagnostic test. Additionally, multi-centre trials suggest the superiority of AMH in comparison to AFC in predicting ovarian response (Iliodromiti et al, 2015).

AFC is not advocated as the sole indicator of ovarian reserve. Conversely, a TV USS offers instantaneous findings and furnishes supplementary insights, such as the detection of ovarian or uterine pathologies, which are crucial for planning future pregnancies within the context of IVF protocols.

7.3 Anti-Müllerian Hormone

AMH, also known as Müllerian-inhibiting substance, is a member of the transforming growth factor-β family. Conveniently, the ovaries are the only source of AMH in women. AMH is produced by granulosa cells of ovarian follicles with expression initiated in small growing primary follicles and declining in the antral stages as follicles gain FSH dependence or become atretic (Durlinger et al, 2002; Weenen et al, 2004).

AMH levels begin increasing from birth, with a distinctive rise in the first few months of life, finally reaching a peak in the mid-20s. Afterwards, there is a steady decline in AMH concentrations until they become undetectable around five years before menopause (Hagen et al, 2010). A slight decrease in AMH concentration, observed around puberty, coincides with the time of maximal follicular recruitment (Nelson et al, 2013). The AMH concentration in serum correlates with the number of antral follicles on ultrasound scans. Relative to other endocrine markers, a decrease in AMH concentration is apparent much earlier on in the approach to menopause. It is beneficial in counselling fertility preservation options since other markers remain static until menopause.

Interestingly, AMH is an accurate measure of ovarian reserve even in women with irregular menstrual cycles, which gives it an advantage over other markers like FSH. In the clinical setting, the serum concentration of AMH is relatively independent of the menstrual cycle. However, some studies have reported significant intra- and inter-cycle fluctuations in AMH concentrations (Melado et al, 2018), suggesting that repeat measurements of AMH can be more dependable. Nevertheless, the consensus is that those fluctuations are too small to affect AMH-guided counselling and clinical decision making in an IVF setting, and AMH measurement at unspecified times in the menstrual cycle is acceptable.

It is worth noting that hormonal contraception users have lower levels of AMH, which recover after its discontinuation. The most prominent decline in AMH levels is seen in the combined contraceptive pill users, with the least impact seen in the intrauterine hormonal device (Hariton et al, 2021). Lowered AMH is the result of changes in follicular dynamics initiated by the prolonged use of exogenous hormones. Although, as mentioned earlier, AMH is produced mainly by small growing follicles, including small pre-antral and antral follicles, the latter are sensitive to gonadotropins, and their number is reduced in women with suppressed pituitary function.

The first developed AMH assay dates back to 1990 and, over the years, has been fraught with difficulties, resulting in an incoherent body of evidence. Initial manual assays lacked precision and reproducibility. Additionally, the results were affected by AMH sample instability and the presence of AMH isoforms leading to significant inter-laboratory variation in AMH results. However, the advent of automated testing offers high reproducibility, strengthening AMH's position as the most accurate biological marker of ovarian reserve.

In preparation for the egg freezing cycle, ovarian reserve testing helps estimate the dose of exogenous gonadotropins needed to stimulate the growth of follicles and successfully retrieve competent oocytes. Women with a low ovarian reserve are likely to under-respond to a standard dose of gonadotrophins. As a result, they may require two or three cycles to obtain a sufficient number of oocytes providing reasonable chances of pregnancy. Knowledge of AMH levels facilitates discussion about the individual approach to the egg freezing cycle, keeping expectations realistic.

On the other end of the spectrum, women with endocrine conditions, like polycystic ovary syndrome, have an elevated risk of over-response, potentially leading to ovarian hyperstimulation syndrome. Women with extremely high AMH concentrations undergoing oocyte freezing risk developing primary ovarian hyperstimulation syndrome. Although self-limiting, it can lead to severe consequences, including ascites, pleural effusion, and thrombosis. New strategies, e.g., utilising the use of agonist trigger to ensure final maturation of oocytes before egg collection as opposed to human chorionic gonadotropin trigger, are well established in clinical practice and have significantly reduced the risk of ovarian hyperstimulation syndrome in this group of patients. Counselling for fertility preservation should therefore routinely include measurements of AMH.

AMH plays a crucial role in planning the fertility preservation cycle, yet the interpretation of its results should invariably incorporate age as a critical factor. Age-related oocyte changes still occur in all older women. Satisfactory or 'normal' AMH levels in the older patient group (above the age of 38) would still not guarantee success in achieving pregnancy even though a 'good' number of oocytes are likely to be harvested.

Ovarian reserve testing is instrumental for clinicians in devising the optimal protocol and determining the appropriate dosage of gonadotropins. An individualised approach to ovarian stimulation medication dosing, anchored in AMH levels, can enhance the safety of the process and diminish the likelihood of cycle cancellation.

7.4 Ovarian Reserve in Young Cancer Patients

Early detection of cancer and improving survival rates have increased life expectancy for young women diagnosed with cancer. However, their quality of life after successful treatment, including the ability to conceive, remains one of the major concerns. Cancer treatment is known to cause a range of severe side effects. Ovaries are particularly sensitive and readily damaged by specific treatment regimens, causing loss of ovarian follicles. Persistent amenorrhoea is an obvious indicator of an effect upon ovarian function. However, the recovery of menses does not imply that the ovarian reserve has been recovered. In many patients, the ovarian reserve becomes significantly reduced, giving them less time to become pregnant and fulfilling their wishes of becoming a mother.

There is a relative paucity of data relating to the specific mechanisms behind chemotherapy/radiotherapy-induced oocyte loss, its extent, potential reversibility, and most importantly, future ability to conceive. The gonadotoxic influence of chemotherapy on ovaries includes effects on both somatic and germ cells and vascular damage. The degree of follicular apoptosis and cortical fibrosis may vary with different types and dosages of chemotherapy. Also, effects upon the pool of primordial follicles may not be the same as on other classes of follicles, e.g., maturing follicles containing dividing granulosa cells. The latter would be the prime target of chemotherapeutic agents as they directly affect actively dividing cells. It is possible that several mechanisms, which could be drug-specific or chemotherapy regimen-specific, take place at the time of exposure and may continue thereafter. Some of the damage may only become evident later. A constant dialogue between somatic cells and germ cells, which is necessary to regulate the growth and maturation of both, may be interrupted, and its re-establishment after profound changes due to chemotherapy exposure may be defective. Based on the mechanism of action and current studies, some agents such as doxorubicin and cyclophosphamide act more on the dividing granulosa cells, while others, such as cisplatin or topoisomerase enzymes, target the oocyte directly (Meirow & Nugent et al, 2001).

The extent of follicular loss would at least partially depend on the size of the ovarian reserve before treatment begins. Testing prior to chemotherapy can allow women to discuss fertility preservation options with the knowledge of their ovarian reserve, anticipated degree of damage and likelihood of future natural pregnancy, all based on the type of chemotherapy and dosage of each agent, which also could be tailored individually according to patients' priorities. AMH characteristics make it particularly applicable in that setting. The other important question is whether women who develop a malignancy have already reduced ovarian reserve, compared to the general population, even before they begin cancer treatment. It could impact the fertility preservation option offered and potential chances of freezing a sufficient number of oocytes.

A prospective cohort study measuring the effect of chemotherapy on ovarian function, assessed by serum AMH, was conducted to address those questions (Palinska-Rudzka et al, 2018). Patients aged 18–43 years with newly diagnosed cancer prior to chemotherapy were recruited from multiple oncology clinics across the UK. A control group was comprised of healthy female volunteers (Figure 7.1). Women with advanced cancer or a history of interventions potentially

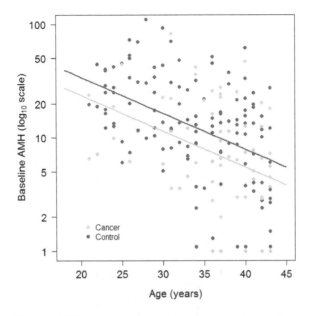

Figure 7.1   Serum AMH concentrations prior to chemotherapy in cancer patients and volunteer groups. Fitted regression model, log-transformed AMH levels (pmol/L). Reproduced with permission from Palinska-Rudzka et al (2018).

impacting ovarian reserve, like previous exposure to gonadotoxic agents/therapies or oophorectomy, were excluded. Serum AMH was measured before any exposure to gonadotoxic agents and at follow-up intervals of 12 months and five years. Healthy volunteers had serum AMH measured at the same intervals.

Additionally, participants completed a detailed questionnaire at the start, one and five years later. In total, 190 women completed the first medical questionnaire, comprising 54 breast cancer patients, 12 lymphoma patients and 124 healthy volunteers. Prior to chemotherapy, there was a significant difference in serum AMH between cancer patients and healthy volunteers (z-test; $p = 0.02$). After adjusting for age and other confounding factors, regression analysis of log-transformed (base 10) AMH showed that serum AMH was 1.4 (95% CI; 1.1 to 1.9) times higher in the healthy volunteers than in the breast and lymphoma group combined (Figure 7.2). Breast cancer

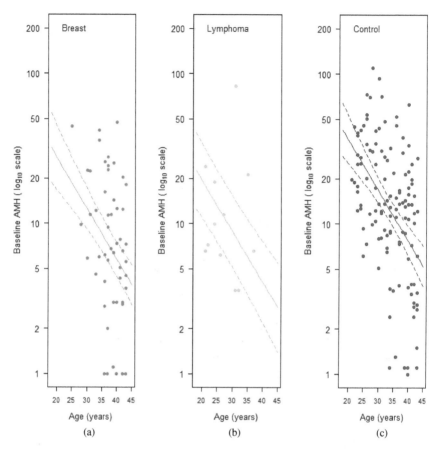

Figure 7.2 Serum AMH concentrations prior to chemotherapy in breast cancer, lymphoma and control groups. A fitted regression model with 95% CI, log-transformed. Reproduced with permission from Palinska-Rudzka et al (2018).

patients had significantly lower AMH than controls, and the trend suggestive of reduced serum AMH in more advanced stages of breast cancer was observed; however, the sample size was small.

Over 90% of breast cancer patients had detectable AMH at one-year follow-up. While serum AMH at one year was low, it remained similar between year one and year five follow-ups, against expected further reduction in AMH levels. It can be explained by ongoing ovarian reserve recovery as disrupted folliculogenesis may take longer to return. In contrast to the breast cancer group, all patients had detectable AMH at one-year and five-year follow-ups in the lymphoma group.

At final follow-up, serum AMH was significantly lower in women who reported amenorrhea over the last ≥12 months compared to those who reported the presence of menstrual cycles, either regular or irregular. However, over 40% of the latter had drastically reduced ovarian reserve, highlighting that the return of menses post-chemotherapy is a poor predictor of fertility potential.

The variation in the rate of follicle loss among individuals is significant, underscoring the limitations of relying on mathematical models for fertility counselling based on age. Consequently, an assessment of the ovarian reserve provides a more precise evaluation of an individual's remaining fertile years, addressing concerns about current and future fertility potential. The role of AMH is particularly prominent in this context, especially for assessing ovarian reserve in female cancer patients considering oocyte cryopreservation. This approach not only enhances the accuracy of fertility assessments but also offers a practical solution for those seeking to preserve their fertility options in challenging circumstances.

References

Broekmans FJ, de Ziegler D, Howles CM, Gougeon A, Trew G, Olivennes F. The antral follicle count: practical recommendations for better standardisation. Fertil Steril. 2010 Aug;94(3):1044–51.

Durlinger AL, Gruijters MJ, Kramer P, Karels B, Ingraham HA, Nachtigal MW, Uilenbroek JT, Grootegoed JA, Themmen AP. Anti-Müllerian hormone inhibits initiation of primordial follicle growth in the mouse ovary. Endocrinology. 2002 Mar;143(3):1076–84.

Evers JL, Slaats P, Land JA, Dumoulin JC, Dunselman GA. Elevated levels of basal estradiol-17beta predict poor response in patients with normal basal levels of follicle-stimulating hormone undergoing in vitro fertilization. Fertil Steril. 1998 Jun;69(6):1010–4.

Faddy MJ, Gosden RG, Gougeon A, Richardson SJ, Nelson JF. Accelerated disappearance of ovarian follicles in mid-life: implications for forecasting menopause. Hum Reprod. 1992 Nov;7(10):1342–6.

Fleming R, Seifer DB, Frattarelli JL, Ruman J. Assessing ovarian response: antral follicle count versus anti-Müllerian hormone. Reprod Biomed Online. 2015 Oct;31(4):486–96.

Hagen CP, Aksglaede L, Sørensen K, Main KM, Boas M, Cleemann L, Holm K, Gravholt CH, Andersson AM, Pedersen AT, Petersen JH, Linneberg A, Kjaergaard S, Juul A. Serum levels of anti-Müllerian hormone as a marker of ovarian function in 926 healthy females from birth to adulthood and in 172 Turner syndrome patients. J Clin Endocrinol Metab. 2010 Nov;95(11):5003–10.

Hariton E, Shirazi TN, Douglas NC, Hershlag A, Briggs SF. Anti-Müllerian hormone levels among contraceptive users: evidence from a cross-sectional cohort of 27,125 individuals. Am J Obstet Gynecol. 2021 Nov;225(5):515.e1–10.

Iliodromiti S, Nelson SM. Ovarian response biomarkers: physiology and performance. Curr Opin Obstet Gynecol. 2015 Jun;27(3):182–6.

Luesley D, Baker P, editors. Obstetrics and gynaecology: an evidence based text for MRCOG. Edward Arnold Publishers; 2004. p. 533–538.

Meirow D, Nugent D. The effects of radiotherapy and chemotherapy on female reproduction. Hum Reprod Update. 2001 Nov-Dec;7(6):535–43.

Melado L, Lawrenz B, Sibal J, Abu E, Coughlan C, Navarro AT, Fatemi HM. Anti-Müllerian hormone during natural cycle presents significant intra and intercycle variations when measured with fully automated assay. Front Endocrinol (Lausanne). 2018 Nov 27;9:686.

Nelson SM. Biomarkers of ovarian response: current and future applications. Fertil Steril. 2013 Mar 15;99(4):963–9.

Palinska-Rudzka KE, Ghobara T, Parsons N, Milner J, Lockwood G, Hartshorne GM. Five-year study assessing the clinical utility of anti-Müllerian hormone measurements in reproductive-age women with cancer. Reprod Biomed Online. 2019 Oct;39(4):712–20.

Razafintsalama-Bourdet M, Bah M, Amand G, Vienet-Lègue L, Pietin-Vialle C, Bry-Gauillard H, Pinto M, Pasquier M, Vernet T, Jung C, Levaillant JM, Massin N. Random antral follicle count performed on any day of the menstrual cycle has the same predictive value as AMH for good ovarian response in IVF cycles. J Gynecol Obstet Hum Reprod. 2022 Jan;51(1):102233.

Wallace WH, Kelsey TW. Human ovarian reserve from conception to the menopause. PLoS One. 2010 Jan 27;5(1):e8772.

Weenen C, Laven JS, Von Bergh AR, Cranfield M, Groome NP, Visser JA, Kramer P, Fauser BC, Themmen AP. Anti-Müllerian hormone expression pattern in the human ovary: potential implications for initial and cyclic follicle recruitment. Mol Hum Reprod. 2004 Feb;10(2):77–83.

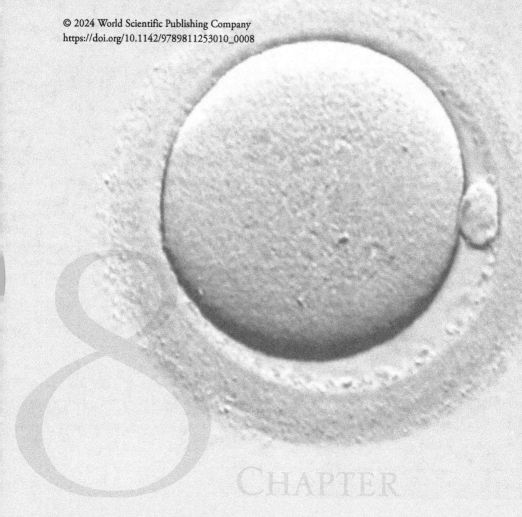

CHAPTER

Clinical Management of Oocyte Vitrification Patients:
Stimulation Protocols and Frozen/Thawed Blastocyst Transfer Protocols

Anabel Salazar Vera and Juan A Garcia-Velasco

8.1 Introduction

The first human pregnancy from a previously cryopreserved oocyte was reported in 1986 (Chen, 1986). Although oocyte cryopreservation has existed for 20 years, the field of fertility preservation (FP) in general has grown hugely in the last two decades. The development of an enabling technology has improved in the past 20 years resulting in widespread clinical practice, mainly because of the vitrification procedure becoming the standard protocol for oocyte cryopreservation.

Despite the great progress made in this field, oocyte cryopreservation was limited to investigational protocols until 2013. The practice committee of the American Society for Reproductive Medicine (ASRM) removed the experimental label from oocyte vitrification that year, stating that oocyte freezing was no more considered as "experimental" and allowed for its routine use in post-menarcheal women facing gonadotoxic therapies (Practice Committees of the American Society for Reproductive Medicine and the Society for Assisted Reproductive Technology, 2013).

However, at that time, the ASRM Practice Committee document did not recommend oocyte cryopreservation for the sole purpose of preventing age-related fertility decline in healthy women, relying on the limited data available about safety, efficacy, ethics, emotional risks, and cost effectiveness. Furthermore, the European Society of Human Reproduction and Embryology (ESHRE) task force on ethics and law concluded that arguments against offering oocyte cryopreservation to women who wish to delay childbirth were not convincing at that time (Dondorp et al, 2012).

In recent years, the use of oocyte cryopreservation has greatly expanded, not only for women facing gonadotoxic treatments but also for other indications, such as delaying childbearing, as well as for the purpose of oocyte donation. Preserving female fertility is crucial in a healthcare system that takes care of patients' future quality of life and general society well-being.

At present, oocyte cryopreservation is recognised by several international scientific societies as the gold standard for FP in post-pubertal women, for both medical and non-medical indications. The main medical indications in addition to cancer diagnoses are gynaecological diseases such as severe endometriosis, systemic diseases compromising the ovarian reserve, and chromosomal or genetic conditions involving premature menopause such as Turner Syndrome and Fragile X Syndrome.

Although women are increasingly seeking to cryopreserve oocytes for age-related fertility loss, named as "planned oocyte cryopreservation", the evidence base remains limited on this indication. Conclusions from the Ethics Committee of the ASRM are that it is an ethically permissible medical treatment that may enhance women's reproductive autonomy and promote social equality, but as with any new treatment, uncertainties exist regarding its efficacy and long-term effects. Thus, practitioners are strongly encouraged to gather and share data to add to scientific understanding about planned oocyte cryopreservation.

8.2 General Considerations for Ovarian Stimulation in Oocyte Vitrification Treatments for Fertility Preservation

Oocyte cryopreservation is a very well-established FP method that requires controlled ovarian stimulation (COS), a clinical procedure widely used in treatments for infertility and recently discussed in the ESHRE Ovarian Stimulation Guideline (Bosch et al, 2020). For the purpose of this chapter on FP, we will focus on the relevant aspects of COS related to patients undergoing FP.

Ovarian stimulation for FP is usually an urgent procedure and that is one of the main reasons for the lack of strong evidence in some of the aspects regarding this field. The collection of a sufficient number of oocytes within a limited time frame is a challenge. From a practical point of view, reproductive medicine specialists should strongly focus on the effectiveness of the procedure and describe the most appropriate strategies to fully optimise the ovarian reserve and maximise the number of oocytes retrieved in the shortest possible time. The evaluation of the ovarian reserve and the selection of an efficient stimulation protocol, as well as oocyte retrieval approach, should be accurately described to maximise the efficacy, efficiency, and safety of the entire procedure.

Assessment of the predicted response to COS is crucial for personalisation of the treatment and to accurately estimate chances of success and inherent risks in addition to complications, such as ovarian hyperstimulation syndrome (OHSS), and potentially increased risks related to the impact of FP in and underlying malign or benign disease in case of oncological purpose of FP.

Thus, the standardisation of COS protocol will be impacted by patient population, and the current chapter will outline options for four populations (Anderson et al, 2020):

- Post-pubertal women diagnosed with cancer undergoing gonadotoxic treatments.
- Post-pubertal women with benign diseases undergoing gonadotoxic treatment (including surgery) or with conditions from which they will lose their fertility prematurely such as endometriosis.
- Transgender patients assigned female at birth.
- Women requesting oocyte cryopreservation due to age-related fertility loss.

Many questions have been raised, particularly those regarding the preferred protocol. Novel approaches have been suggested for specific patient groups, such as random-start ovarian stimulation, and ovarian stimulation in the context of oestrogen-sensitive diseases.

8.3 Ovarian Stimulation in Cancer Patients Undergoing Fertility Preservation Treatment

8.3.1 Preferred Protocol

When we stimulate the ovaries to produce a multi-follicular development, a fast rising of oestradiol levels occurs, and this setback may trigger a premature luteinising hormone surge. In order to avoid this situation and to ensure that follicles may grow sufficiently large to obtain the best-quality oocytes, the use of agents that block the gonadotropin-releasing hormone (GnRH) pulse signal will contribute to an efficient ovarian stimulation procedure. In general, in most of *in vitro* fertilisation/intracytoplasmic sperm injection (IVF/ICSI) cycles, according to the evidence shown in the last ESHRE Guidelines for Ovarian Stimulation (Bosch et al, 2020), GnRH antagonist protocol is recommended over the GnRH agonist protocols given the comparable efficacy and higher safety in the general population. Although the first studies reported slight and lower pregnancy rates, which delayed the implementation of the GnRH antagonist protocol, several large meta-analyses published in the past 5–7 years support similar live birth rates, such as the evidence from a Cochrane meta-analysis including 73 randomised controlled trials (RCTs), comparing the GnRH antagonist protocol with the long GnRH agonist protocol (Al-Inany et al, 2016), obtaining no difference in live birth rates (12 RCT, odds ratio 1.02, 95% confidence interval 0.85–1.23, 2303 women). Moreover, lower OHSS rate in women who received GnRH antagonist compared with those treated with GnRH agonist is also reported in this publication (6% (290/4474) vs 11% (396/3470); 36 RCT, odds ratio 0.61, 95% confidence interval 0.51–0.72, 7944 women).

Later RCTs published after the meta-analysis showed similar results in terms of pregnancy OHSS rates in the antagonist group. Regarding the moment of introduction of the GnRH antagonist during stimulation, no differences in terms of cycle outcomes have been shown between a fixed (day 6) compared to flexible (leading follicle of 14 mm) protocol.

Focusing on our target group for FP, evidence in the ESHRE Guideline on Ovarian Stimulation and Female Fertility Preservation strongly recommends the GnRH antagonist protocol for COS in women seeking FP for medical reasons due to its feasibility in urgent situations, short time and safety reasons. This recommendation is based on the publications from two systematic reviews including a total of 33 studies (Boots et al, 2016; Rodgers et al, 2017) and 14 other investigations reported in this guideline (Anderson et al, 2020). They reported data on cancer patients undergoing COS for oocyte and/or embryo cryopreservation in more than 2200 cycles, 90% of them performed with GnRH antagonist protocols. They included patients following random-start ovarian stimulation, as well as the use of aromatase inhibitors or tamoxifen in women with breast cancer. Different trigger types at the final oocyte maturation were used. The main outcome measure was usually the overall number of oocytes obtained and the number of mature oocytes among them. Limited data on embryo replacement and live birth are available.

The use of GnRH antagonist protocol allows shortening the duration of stimulation and triggering oocyte maturation with a GnRH agonist is possible in this type of cycle. This option will reduce the risk of OHSS in high-responder women and should be the standard option for this kind of patients, taking into consideration that most of them will shortly start treatment such as chemo/radiotherapy or surgery.

Further, in cancer patients, who are at higher risk of thrombosis due to their oncologic status, antagonist protocol seems to be preferred since they enable GnRH agonist trigger, therefore reducing the risk of OHSS.

Due to its feasibility and safety the antagonist protocol should be planned for every patient undergoing FP, even social egg freezing.

8.3.2 Random Start Protocol

In patients with cancer, concerns about COS must be ruled out, such as the delay in starting chemotherapy. If we follow conventional COS, initiating at the beginning of the follicular phase, COS may require up to six weeks to conclude. Thus, in urgent FP cycles, random-start COS is an option. Random-start ovarian stimulation, which means initiating COS immediately and independently of the menstrual cycle, has become an efficient option in FP strategies, allowing accomplishment of oocyte retrieval in no more than two weeks in most cases. While the evidence indicates that oocyte competence is probably not impacted if COS is started in the luteal phase compared to the follicular phase, there are still insufficient data on live birth rates to confirm strongly its role in ovarian stimulation for FP. There is still lack of evidence due to the few studies available. The drug marketing approval for gonadotropin use in luteal phase needs to be considered according to the conclusion from the ESHRE Guideline Group on Ovarian Stimulation (Anderson et al, 2020). Accordingly, from the current evidence available, random-start ovarian stimulation is probably not recommended for the general population in terms of safety and efficacy compared to the standard early follicular phase stimulation, and there is also no difference in terms of number of oocytes retrieved. Moreover, freeze-all oocytes or embryos is mandatory in this protocol.

The systematic review from Boots et al (2016), including eight non-randomised studies, six of which were in a context of FP, showed in 251 women that COS cycles starting in the luteal phase were slightly longer and required higher doses of gonadotrophins comparing with standard stimulation performed in the follicular phase. There was no significant difference in peak serum oestradiol levels comparing both protocols, and oocytes from the cycles initiated in the luteal phase were more efficient in fertilisation rates.

After the ESHRE Guideline publication, we have a few articles regarding the efficacy of random-start protocol for FP but they do not elucidate any difference on their results, such as the one from Cavagna et al (2018). They reported similar outcomes regarding number of oocytes retrieved and maturity rates. They also found that significant higher follicle-stimulating hormone (FSH) or human menopausal gonadotropins (hMG) dose were required in cycles starting in the luteal phase.

This issue was also reported in Maklund et al (2020), in a prospective study of FP in women with breast cancer reported on 380 cycles using a GnRH antagonist regimen. They compared 201 cycles with 179 cases of conventional start in women with breast cancer. The use of random start was not associated with the number of retrieved oocytes and the number of cryopreserved oocytes (9.0 [range 0–24] vs 10.6 [range 0–40]) and embryos (4.8 [range 0–29] vs 4.8 [range 0–16]) were similar between the groups. Random start group required a higher total dose of gonadotropins (p < 0.001).

In conclusion, both cost but also safety studies should be carried out, because non-conventional stimulation requires the use of higher FSH dose and long-term child health follow-up must be performed according to the modified hormonal environment of the oocytes used in this kind of protocol.

Current recommendations from the ESHRE Guideline are not strongly supporting late luteal phase start of gonadotropins for poor responders and similarly early luteal phase start of gonadotropins is probably not recommended for normal and poor responders.

Quality of evidence is low and non-consistent on the use of luteal start of FSH in normal and poor responders, and no data is available from polycystic ovary syndrome patients.

Because of the mandatory use of freeze-all of oocytes and embryos needed in this kind of protocol, it may be an option in non-transfer cycles. Therefore, luteal phase stimulation could be considered as an option in specific cases for organisation and shortened time to oocyte retrieval, for example in urgent oncologic FP, which is the aim of this chapter, as well as in freeze-all policy programs.

8.3.3 Double Stimulation

Double stimulation in the same cycle, also called "dual stimulation", "DuoStim" (Vaiarelli et al, 2018) or the "Shanghai protocol" involves two stimulation protocols within the same ovarian cycle. This is particularly suited for oncological patients with poor prognosis, who require maximising of the availability of their ovarian reserve in a limited time.

Due to the extremely dynamic nature of follicular development this kind of protocol has emerged in recent years. The classic theory of single recruitment episode may lead to the grow of a single cohort of antral follicles in the follicular phase of the ovarian cycle after luteal regression. But this theory has been overtaken by the evidence that multiple waves arise during an ovarian cycle in many mammals. Such evidence was confirmed in humans leading to the definition of the wave theory, according to which 2–3 cohorts of antral follicles are recruited per ovarian cycle. DuoStim combines a conventional follicular phase stimulation with luteal phase stimulation. The second cycle is performed immediately after the oocyte first pick-up. So, two pick-ups will be performed in approximately two weeks. It allows one to obtain more oocytes in a shorter time period.

The first publication with double stimulation was reported by Kuang et al (2014) who showed that COS with this specific protocol results in the retrieval of oocytes with similar developmental competence.

As shown in luteal phase stimulation protocols, the quality of oocytes retrieved in this second cycle seems to be as good as the ones coming from the first stimulation, with the same euploid embryo rate reported by Vaiarelli et al (2018).

There are no studies comparing the results from double stimulation with two consecutive conventional stimulations, although current evidence shows that double stimulation is feasible, providing sufficient quality of eggs. Randomised controlled studies are needed to assess the advantages and disadvantages of double stimulation compared to conventional protocols.

New options for ovarian stimulation improvement in terms of efficiency and efficacy are arising, especially in urgent FP cycles. This is based on studies that have reported more oocytes with double stimulation compared to follicular phase stimulation and comparable pregnancy rates from oocytes obtained in the luteal or follicular phase. The disadvantage of mandatory freeze-all procedure resulting from luteal start stimulation is irrelevant in the context of FP.

8.3.4 Anti-oestrogen Therapies

FP in breast cancer represents a complex issue since the disease is linked in many cases with tumours that are considered oestrogen sensitive. Furthermore, ovarian stimulation with the aim to obtain oocytes or embryos to be frozen results in supra-physiological serum oestradiol levels. Although temporary, this side effect of higher oestradiol levels could theoretically result in the proliferation of malignant cells. Despite this fact, there are no data demonstrating an adverse effect of ovarian stimulation for FP in women with breast cancer.

In an effort to reduce the potential harm associated with high oestradiol levels, innovative stimulation protocols have been developed, including the use of aromatase inhibitors such as letrozole (Oktay et al, 2010). It is frequently used during stimulation and maintained for a few days after oocyte retrieval. This combination may minimise oestrogen exposure and will reduce systemic oestradiol levels as previously reported by Oktay et al (2005). Cycles using letrozole may be also potentially safer for women with endometrial hyperplasia or borderline ovarian tumours. The addition of letrozole to ovarian stimulation has also been proposed for patient groups where systemic oestradiol increase is not desirable, such as transgender men and patients with increased inherent thrombosis risk.

The existing quality of evidence concerning ovarian stimulation for FP in women with oestrogen-sensitive cancer is still low given the number and quality of studies available. Most of the publications are observational studies, with a small number of patients, and a relatively short duration of their follow-up. Strong evidence regarding the safety of ovarian stimulation in women with diagnosis of breast cancer would require long-term and large-scale studies, which still do not yet exist.

In conclusion, ovarian stimulation for FP in oestrogen-sensitive diseases and the concomitant use of anti-oestrogen therapy, such as letrozole, can be considered. However, the use of letrozole is off label for ovarian stimulation and safety concerns have been raised regarding possible teratogenicity associated with letrozole, according to the evidence raised on the last ESHRE Guidelines (Bosch et al, 2020; Anderson et al, 2020).

8.4 Ovarian Stimulation for Fertility Preservation in Transgender Men

Transgender individuals present with a gender identity that is incongruent with their phenotypic sex assigned at birth. Transgender men are assigned female at birth and usually identify as male. Gender dysphoria is a condition in which a person experiences internal psychological conflict due to incongruence of his/her gender assigned at birth and the gender with which he/she identifies. The estimated prevalence of adults who identify as 'transgender' or 'gender nonconforming' in the USA is 0.6% of the population. Despite an increasing focus on transgender health research, gender-nonconforming youth and young adults remain an under-served population that is seen more often by health care professionals generally and in fertility clinics.

Some transgender individuals suffering from gender dysphoria might need gender-affirming medical intervention in order to masculinise body parts to alleviate the gender dysphoria. Gender-affirming medical intervention could include sex reassignment surgery and/or cross-sex hormonal treatment. Although these treatment options often succeed in reducing such symptoms, they can also negatively impact future reproductive potential. For example, among transgender men, gender-affirming medical intervention will lead to irreversible infertility in the case of hysterectomy and oophorectomy. Moreover, masculinising hormone therapy (androgens) alone may have an atrophic effect on the endometrium or cause hyperplasia of the ovarian cortex and stroma. Although there is evidence of effects on reproductive organs from gender-affirming hormone therapy, the effect on actual fertility, and the reversibility of such effects, is currently unknown.

Studies investigating aspects of FP in connection with gender dysphoria are rare. One study in Belgium among 50 transgender men showed that half of them wanted to have children at the time of the study, and if FP options had been available at the time of their transition, 38% would have considered using it.

Transgender individuals should be offered FP aimed to store oocytes prior to starting gender-affirming therapy, both because of the current lack of knowledge on fertility after hormone therapy and to possibly prevent reoccurrence of gender dysphoria following transition. FP options are the same for transgender individuals as cisgender individuals, requiring transvaginal ultrasound examinations and ovarian stimulation with gonadotropins. These interventions may have a negative impact on gender dysphoria, becoming a challenge for this patient group and their medical team. Successful management requires sensitivity and awareness of these issues. Patients should be informed that ovarian stimulation will increase their serum oestradiol levels, and that transvaginal ultrasound monitoring may be necessary. Strategies to decrease this distress include the concomitant use of aromatase inhibitors during stimulation to minimise oestradiol elevations, which has already been shown not to compromise outcomes in breast cancer patients undergoing ovarian stimulation for FP (Armuand et al, 2017).

In some cases, patients may agree to temporary discontinue their cross-sex hormonal treatment to undergo ovarian stimulation aiming at oocyte vitrification. The use of long-term testosterone treatment, in certain cases with treatment with a GnRH agonist, may result in the patients being severely downregulated and hypogonadotropic, comparable to women on long-term GnRH agonist treatment for endometriosis. Discontinuation of testosterone treatment prior to ovarian stimulation for FP in transgender men has been reported, using antagonist protocols. In the first study from Adeleye et al (2019) they compare ovarian stimulation and pregnancy outcomes between transgender men with and without a history of testosterone use to cisgender women. 13 transgender men following ovarian stimulation, seven who had discontinued treatment with testosterone, were compared with six without previous treatment with testosterone. Time from stopping testosterone was not reported. There were no differences in the baseline follicle count, cycle length, or FSH and hMG used. Fewer oocytes were retrieved in patients with previous testosterone use (12 interquartile range [4–26]) vs 25.5 [18–28]). In another report from Leung et al (2019), assisted reproductive technology outcomes in a female-to-male transgender cohort were compared with those of a matched cisgender cohort. 19 transgender men underwent cycles for oocyte or embryo cryopreservation, and seven underwent cycles with embryos transferred. Over 60% of the patients had been on treatment with testosterone (range 3 months – 17 years). All patients stopped testosterone before cycle starts (average 4 months, range 1–12 months) and almost all resumed resumption of menses and had normal baseline FSH, anti-Müllerian hormone and oestradiol levels at cycle start. A similar number of oocytes were retrieved, and peak oestradiol levels were found to be comparable to cisgender women undergoing treatment for infertility. Ovarian stimulation protocol was determined by the treating physician. Almost all used an antagonist stimulation protocol, whereby dosing of gonadotropins was adjusted according to standard protocol in relation to the individual's response. These protocols were the same as those used for cisgender patients.

To summarise, the main recommendations of the ESHRE Guidelines for Fertility Preservation (Anderson et al, 2020) are:

- For ovarian stimulation in transgender men aiming at oocyte cryopreservation, GnRH antagonist protocols can be considered as they have been shown to be feasible and with numbers of oocytes retrieved comparable to those obtained in cisgender women when individuals have stopped previous treatment with testosterone.
- The addition of letrozole to the antagonist protocol can be considered as it may enhance treatment adherence for transgender men by reducing estrogenic symptoms.
- Published data on ovarian stimulation in transgender men are limited to small case series, but show feasibility of ovarian stimulation, even in patients that have previously used testosterone treatments.

8.5 Ovarian Stimulation for Fertility Preservation for Medical Reasons Other Than Cancer: Endometriosis

Endometriosis is a chronic disorder that affects approximately 175 million people, and 6% to 10% of women in their fertile years. Furthermore, endometriosis is a situation in which women are at risk of significant loss in ovarian reserve, due to the progress of the disease or the need for ovarian surgery, especially in its severe forms. This issue results in a poor reproductive outcome after IVF. The current therapeutic approaches are far from being curative, making these patients suitable candidates for FP, especially when surgical excision of the ovarian endometrioma is performed.

Oocyte vitrification is currently considered an efficient option for elective FP in women of reproductive age. Endometriosis is indeed one of those conditions that may be potentially considered as beneficiaries of FP. The discussion revolves around the limited information regarding the efficiency of FP in this particular population and lack of evidence of the quantity and quality of the oocytes retrieved, leading to its generalised use still remaining controversial.

A recent study from Cobo et al (2020) concluded that FP gives patients with endometriosis a valid treatment option to help them increase their reproductive chances, suggesting that performing surgery after ovarian stimulation for FP in young women will be beneficial for this indication. The study included 485 women diagnosed with endometriosis who returned to use their oocytes after 1.7 years of storage for FP and reported the birth of 225 healthy babies. They collected the oocytes with mean age 35.7 years. Antagonist and agonist protocols were used for ovarian stimulation. The initial dose of gonadotropins was selected based on patient age, body mass index, and the assessment of ovarian reserve based on antral follicle count and/or (more recently) anti-Müllerian hormone levels.

In the antagonist protocol, COS was initiated on Day 2 or 3 of a spontaneous cycle. An initial dose of 225–300 IU recombinant FSH and 75–150 IU highly purified hMG was administered until triggering. When a leading follicle reached ≥14 mm, a GnRH antagonist was administered at 0.25 mg/day. Final oocyte maturation was triggered with a single dose of a GnRH agonist when the mean diameter of two follicles was ≥18 mm. In some cases, triggering was performed with 250 μg of recombinant hCG. Oocyte retrieval was scheduled 36 h later. In some cases, clomiphene was added to the antagonist protocol at a daily dose of 50–100 mg for 5 days, initiated on Days 2–3 of the cycle, and combined with 150–300 IU of hMG from Day 3 and every other day until triggering.

For the agonist protocol, the GnRH agonist (0.1 mg/day) was initiated on Day 21 of the previous cycle (long protocol). On Day 3 of the menstrual cycle, recombinant FSH and hMG were administered as in the antagonist protocol. Ovulation was induced by administering recombinant hCG (250 µg) following the same criteria of number and follicle sizes. In some cases, COS was initiated on Day 1 or 2 of a spontaneous cycle by administering the GnRH agonist (0.2 mg/24 h). From Day 3 onward, the dose was adjusted to 0.1 mg/24 h and gonadotropins started being administered.

Accordingly, in the younger group of women aged under 35 years, the oocyte survival, implantation, pregnancy, and cumulative live birth rates were statistically significantly lower for the group of endometriosis patients than for the young elective FP women. A lower oocyte yield, as well as worse clinical results, were observed when they made the comparison between patients aged 35 years and women over 35 years.

In a second study from the same group (Cobo et al, 2021) they analysed how the number of oocytes used affect the cumulative live birth rate in endometriosis patients who had their oocytes vitrified for FP. It was a retrospective observational study including data from 485 women from the previous study in 2020. A total of 260 patients were aged ≤35 years old while the remaining 225 were older than 35. Stages I–II of endometriosis were diagnosed by laparoscopy, while deep infiltrating stages III–IV were confirmed by ultrasound in non-surgical patients. The question about the number of oocytes to vitrify for assessing success rates was crucial, and this question becomes more relevant in endometriosis patients, and besides the number, it is important to take into consideration that oocytes in endometriosis patients may have worse quality as previously reported from other groups. Their results show that the cumulative live birth rate increased as the number of oocytes used per patient was higher, reaching 89.5% using 22 eggs. Better outcomes were observed in young women, with 95.4% cumulative live birth rate in the group under 35 years old using 20 oocytes versus 79.6% in the older women.

In conclusion, the probability of live birth increases as the number of oocytes used increases in patients with endometriosis, and better outcomes were observed among young women.

8.5.1 Progestin-primed Ovarian Stimulation for Fertility Preservation in Endometriosis Patients

Several ovarian stimulation protocols originally developed for assisted reproductive technology have been used for FP, especially for women with cancer. Recently, Kuang et al (2015) described a progestin-primed ovarian stimulation (PPOS) protocol using exogenous progesterone to replace the GnRH agonist or antagonist in the follicular phase. No significant difference regarding number of mature oocytes retrieved and number of frozen embryos was showed from the PPOS protocol compared with the standard antagonist one. Indeed, there is still a scarcity of evidence in assessing the most effective stimulation protocol in the context of endometriosis patients.

In a recent study from Mathieu et al (2020) they found that antagonist and PPOS protocols were associated with similar results but the cost-effectiveness analysis was in favour of PPOS protocols. They conducted a prospective cohort study associated with a cost-effectiveness analysis, where the main outcomes were the number of retrieved and vitrified oocytes, and direct medical costs. They included 108 women with endometriosis who had a single stimulation cycle performed with either an antagonist or a PPOS protocol. Patients on long-term oral progestin treatment who enrolled in the antagonist protocol stopped progestin treatment and the protocol started on the first or second day of a natural cycle. For the PPOS protocol, patients could continue their long-term oral progestin treatment and start the protocol when they wished. Patients in the PPOS protocol without long-term oral progestin treatment started an oral treatment by desogestrel at the same time as ovarian stimulation, on the first day of a natural cycle. In both groups, gonadotropin (150/450 UI FSH or hMG) was injected daily according to body mass index, anti-Müllerian hormone and antral follicle count. In the antagonist protocol group, a GnRH antagonist was injected daily from Day 6 to the trigger day. When three dominant follicles reached 18 mm in diameter, the final stage of oocyte maturation was triggered with the use of 0.2 mg triptorelin or Ovitrelle® 250 μg. Oocyte retrieval was performed 34–36 h after the trigger. No differences were observed between the protocols in terms of duration of the stimulation, the total dose of gonadotropin, and the number of consultations. The results from the study highlighted that antagonist and PPOS protocols are associated with similar outcomes in terms of number of retrieved and vitrified oocytes with a cost analysis in favour of PPOS protocols.

8.6 Ovarian Stimulation for Fertility Preservation in Patients with Age-related Fertility Decline

Egg freezing for age-related fertility loss is increasing and has largely replaced embryo cryopreservation as a fertility option for women without a male partner. Women going into this process are young and healthy and they do not usually have pre-existing medical problems. International guidelines generally support oocyte cryopreservation for age-related fertility loss but recommend that it should be used with caution. This is causing some controversy and the ethical acceptability has been widely debated. Regarding what is the preferred stimulation protocol for FP for social reasons, we need to focus on the main critical outcomes which are collecting the maximum number of oocytes possible and preventing OHSS and other complications.

According to the ESHRE Guidelines for Ovarian Stimulation (Bosch et al, 2020) GnRH antagonist protocols are preferred since they shorten the duration of ovarian stimulation, offer the possibility of triggering final oocyte maturation with GnRH agonist in case of high ovarian response, and reduce the risk of OHSS.

The quality of evidence about the use of random start protocols is still low on this topic. Evidence indicates that oocyte competence is probably not impacted by its luteal phase origin compared to follicular phase. Absence of adverse effects on neonatal outcomes and long-term child health need to be evaluated on a larger scale. As we are discussing healthy patients going through this treatment to preserve their eggs for a future process, we are usually able to decide the best time in the cycle to start stimulating, so in our opinion there is no really strong evidence to support the random start protocol while results are still lacking.

For ovarian stimulation for FP in oestrogen-sensitive diseases the concomitant use of anti-oestrogen therapy, such as letrozole, can be considered. Due to the fact that letrozole is still an off-label alternative we should try to avoid its use in FP for age-related fertility loss.

8.7 Efficacy and Safety of Ovarian Stimulation in Fertility Preservation

8.7.1 The use of Progestins for Pituitary Suppression During Ovarian Stimulation Compared with Standard Protocols

As previously described in endometriosis patients, progestins can present an effective option for women who do not contemplate a fresh embryo transfer, which include our target FP patients in this chapter. A comprehensive and systematic review including meta-analyses carried out by Ata et al (2021) showed that duration of stimulation, gonadotrophin consumption and oocyte yield were similar with progestins and GnRH analogues. 10 studies were included comparing progestins with GnRH antagonists, six with GnRH agonists and six with other progestins or different dosages of the same progestin. Sensitivity analyses suggested that progestins were associated with significantly lower gonadotrophin consumption than the long GnRH agonist protocol, and significantly higher gonadotrophin consumption than the short GnRH agonist protocol. Studies comparing medroxyprogesterone acetate, dydrogesterone and micronised progesterone suggested similar ovarian response and pregnancy outcomes. The euploidy status of embryos from progestin-primed cycles was similar to that of embryos from conventional stimulation cycles. Avoiding GnRH analogue injections and taking progestin pills are assumed to be more convenient for the patients. Different routes of administration for progestins, for example vaginal or transdermal, can be investigated. Although it seems to be an appropriate option for ovarian stimulation in FP, more information on the course of future pregnancies, obstetrics and prenatal outcomes, as well as neonatal and long-term infant data including health and children development, are still needed.

8.7.2 Is the Addition of Hormonal Assessment to Ultrasound Monitoring Improving Efficacy and Safety?

A Cochrane meta-analysis on monitoring of ovarian stimulation in IVF/ICSI with ultrasound alone compared to ultrasound plus serum oestradiol concentration combining six RCTs, including 781 women, conducted by Kwan et al, did not appear to reduce the probability of OHSS, nor increase the probability of clinical pregnancy or the number of oocytes retrieved. The recommendation from ESHRE Guidelines is that the addition of oestradiol measurements to ultrasound monitoring is not superior to monitoring by ultrasound alone in terms of efficacy and safety.

Similar conclusions are expected for the use of a hormonal panel of oestradiol, progesterone and luteinising hormone measurements in combination with ultrasound monitoring. The addition of hormonal assessments is not improving the number of oocytes retrieved according to two studies described in the ESHRE Guideline for Ovarian Stimulation.

8.7.3 General Risks of Ovarian Stimulation

In studies of FP for cancer patients, usually we need a period of two weeks to obtain oocytes after ovarian stimulation and oocyte retrieval.

This seems to be an acceptable time frame from diagnosis and starting of cancer therapy in most cases.

FP cycles should be performed only in women with no contraindication for ovarian stimulation and/or oocyte pick-up, as these risks are related with the altered endocrine environment generated by the gonadotrophin treatment, which may increase the risk for thrombosis. Haemorrhage and infections are potential risks considered in all cases. The risk for a thrombotic complication may be increased in women with certain diseases including malignant conditions in general, and autoimmune or rare diseases.

Patients suffering from diseases featuring low platelet counts or lymphopenia may present with inherently higher risks of bleeding and/or infection following transvaginal puncture procedures for oocyte pick-up.

The potential risk of OHSS should be considered in all patients, not only in FP for cancer, but in particular for young or expected high responder patients. OHSS should be avoided in women undergoing FP for medical reasons due to the increased risks of complications such as thrombosis. Furthermore, OHSS may delay a planned cancer treatment, which will be a negative side effect we need to especially avoid. It has been established in large studies that the risk of OHSS increases when >15 oocytes are collected (Bosch et al, 2020). In order to perform a safe protocol for FP patients and following recommendation from the ESHRE Guidelines (Bosch et al, 2020) a GnRH agonist trigger is strongly recommended for final oocyte maturation in women at risk of OHSS.

8.7.4 Frozen/Thawed Blastocyst Transfer Protocol

Although there is an evident increased demand for FP both for elective and oncological purposes in recent years, very little evidence about the outcome of these cycles in the FP population is available in the literature. It is crucial to be aware of the success rates after using frozen oocytes; the largest series published to date was conducted by Cobo et al (2018). It is a retrospective, observational multicentre study with 6362 women that went to vitrification cycles for FP and the warming cycles of women who returned to attempt pregnancy from January 2007 to May 2018. The endometrial preparation for embryo transfer was hormone substitution therapy with oral oestradiol valerate, 6 mg per day. Approximately 10 days after, serum oestradiol levels and endometrial thickness were assessed. After that, administration of micronised progesterone 800 mg/day vaginally was initiated three days prior to an embryo transfer for Day 3, and five days prior to embryo transfer on blastocyst stage. If pregnancy was achieved, administration of oestradiol valerate and progesterone was maintained until gestation week 12. This report shows the largest series to date, with more than 6000 women performing over 8000 FP cycles, of whom approximately 700 have returned to attempt pregnancy, and with 162 and 25 healthy babies born in the Endometriosis-FP group and the Onco-FP group, respectively. They observed poorer outcomes in cancer patients compared to the age-matched Endometriosis-FP women, though the hypothetical effect of the presence of cancer on survival and the cumulative live birth rate was not statistically confirmed. The fewer cancer patients returning to use their oocytes may explain the lack of confirmation of the impact of the disease on reproductive outcomes.

Regarding the scarce information about the outcomes, we may focus on how we perform endometrial preparations for standard patients in the IVF process, and try to understand if there is any benefit from one protocol to another. The main question should be if the type of endometrial preparation will be a factor affecting the outcomes, taking into consideration that in the onco-fertility group some patients may have stopped their cycles due to the oncological treatment, or others may have received also radiotherapy affecting pelvis structure. Adequate hormonal preparation of the endometrium is of utmost importance for frozen embryo replacement cycles to provide optimal chances of pregnancy in general population patients, and also for fresh donor cycles which follow similar endometrium preparation protocols.

Many drugs and different types of administration have been tried by several investigators in order to optimise implantation rates and improve the success rates of the embryo transfer procedures. Some of the options are: stimulated cycles (to produce endogenous oestradiol), programmed cycles (using exogenous oestradiol) and natural cycles (allowing the ovaries to produce oestradiol without stimulation). Furthermore, avoiding spontaneous ovulation with GnRH agonists and antagonists could have some impact, and using other drugs such as aspirin or steroids that could potentially enhance the endometrial receptivity were also evaluated.

All these issues have been presented in a recent Cochrane systematic review conducted by Glujovsky et al (2020). They analysed 31 RCTs (5426 women included) evaluating endometrial preparation in women undergoing fresh donor cycles and frozen embryo transfers. They analysed RCTs comparing different interventions such as the dose and route of administration of oestrogens and progestogen, the use of drugs that stop the patient from ovulating prematurely (GnRH agonists), and the use of other medications to improve the endometrium.

They concluded that there is insufficient evidence on the use of any particular intervention for endometrial preparation in women undergoing fresh donor cycles and frozen embryo transfers.

Some of the key results from this review are:

- An improvement in live birth in a stimulated cycle (with letrozole) compared to a programmed cycle remains uncertain. The impact on miscarriage rate and endometrial thickness remains uncertain. A stimulated cycle may improve clinical pregnancy rate but there is insufficient data about multiple pregnancy cycle cancellation and other adverse effects.
- The impact of natural cycle vs programmed cycle improvement on live birth rate, pregnancy rate, miscarriage rate and endometrial thickness remains unclear.
- An uncertain improvement from the use of transdermal oestrogens compared with oral on clinical pregnancy rate and miscarriage rate has been found.

- Starting progesterone on the day of the donor oocyte retrieval or the day after (Day 0 or Day 1) increases the clinical pregnancy rate and probably reduces cycle cancellation rate.
- A cycle with GnRH agonist compared to a cycle without it may improve live birth rate but there is no evidence that one GnRH agonist is better than other. However, the use of GnRH antagonists compared to agonists probably improves clinical pregnancy rate.
- The use of aspirin remains uncertain in the improvement on live birth rate, clinical pregnancy rate or endometrial thickness. There is insufficient evidence supporting the use of steroids compared to a cycle without steroids.

More studies are needed to better understand which is the best protocol for endometrial preparation for frozen embryo transfer.

Another systematic review on the topic from Mumusoglu et al (2021) highlighted an interesting topic concerning the variation in serum progesterone levels not previously described in the Cochrane review. In their systematic review of the topic, they aimed to compare different frozen embryo transfer protocols in terms of reproductive, obstetric and maternal outcomes as follows:

Hormone Replacement Treatment (HRT)

HRT with GnRH agonist suppression

HRT without GnRH agonist suppression

True Natural Cycle (t-NC)

t-NC with luteal phase support

t-NC without luteal phase support

Modified Natural Cycle (m-NC)

m-NC with luteal phase support

m-NC without luteal phase support

Mild Ovarian Stimulation

clomiphene citrate/aromatase inhibitor (letrozole)/FSH

HRT and NC are the most commonly used protocols. In the HRT cycle, suppression of follicular growth, endometrial proliferation and subsequent secretory transformation are achieved by the timely administration of exogenous oestradiol and progesterone. In NC, however, endogenous oestradiol and progesterone secreted in a spontaneous cycle will prime the endometrium.

In HRT cycle, oestradiol priming with oral or transdermal protocol has similar efficacy. The optimal duration for oestradiol priming is between 10 and 36 days, without compromising reproductive outcomes. Pituitary suppression with GnRH agonist decreases the cycle cancelation rate; indeed, HRT without suppression is more patient friendly and is associated with similar outcomes when compared with those performed with GnRH agonist suppression.

Regarding progesterone administration researchers concluded that there is scarce data on the impact of different routes (vaginal, intramuscular, subcutaneous, oral or rectal routes) on reproductive outcome in HRT cycles. Vaginal administration is the most commonly used option. Future studies are needed to confirm the optimum dosing of different vaginal intakes of progesterone. Since there is no corpus luteum in HRT cycles, progesterone should be continued until the 10th to 12th weeks of gestation.

Regarding the day of starting progesterone administration, there is paucity of data on the impact of the length of the progesterone exposure on the reproductive outcome. The limited evidence suggests that, for the optimal length of progesterone exposure before frozen embryo transfer, Day 3 embryos should be transferred on the third or fourth day of progesterone administration and Day 5/6 blastocysts on the fifth or sixth day of progesterone administration. A higher live birth rate for Day 6 vitrified blastocysts when transferred on the seventh day of progesterone administration, as reported by a single retrospective study, should be warranted by further RCTs.

Referring to NC, we must differentiate between t-NC and m-NC which should be performed in patients with regular menstrual cycles.

In t-NC, to schedule frozen embryo transfer, the timing of spontaneous ovulation needs to be accurately confirmed, which means frequent endocrine and transvaginal ultrasonographic monitoring. Therefore, it is less flexible when compared with HRT and m-NC. In m-NC, triggering is performed when the leading follicle is between 16–20 mm in diameter and scheduling is performed accordingly. m-NC also requires less endocrine and ultrasonographic monitoring when compared with t-NC and, consequently, is considered more patient friendly. In t-NC cycles, differences in definition of luteinising hormone surge may result in differences in timing of frozen embryo transfer which may have impact on reproductive outcomes. Clearly the optimal definition of luteinising hormone surge associated with the best reproductive outcome should be explored.

8.7.5 The Impact of Low Serum Progesterone: Rescue Protocols in Hormone Replacement Treatment Endometrial Preparation

A natural question to ask regarding patients with low serum progesterone levels is whether the cycle can be "rescued" with additional exogenous progesterone, using the same or a different route of administration, and if there is any serum progesterone threshold on the day of embryo transfer in HRT preparation cycles below which the chances of ongoing pregnancy are reduced. This was analysed by Labarta et al (2021) in a recent publication based on a previous study where they found that serum progesterone levels <9.2 ng/ml on the day of embryo transfer significantly decreased ongoing pregnancy rates in a sample of 211 oocyte donation recipients. In the new study, they assessed whether these results were applicable to all infertile patients under an artificial endometrial preparation cycle, regardless of the oocyte origin.

This was a prospective cohort study that enrolled 1205 patients scheduled for embryo transfer after an artificial endometrial preparation cycle with oestradiol valerate and micronised vaginal progesterone

(400 mg twice daily). They identified a threshold of serum progesterone as 8.8 ng/ml on the day of embryo transfer for these patients, in cycles with own or donated oocytes. One-third of patients receiving progesterone at this dose showed inadequate levels of serum progesterone.

Further RCTs are clearly warranted, exploring different types and routes of progesterone to establish the success of the rescue protocol. Finally, the lowest serum progesterone level suitable for rescue should also be defined.

References

Adeleye AJ, Cedars MI, Smith J, Mok-Lin E. Ovarian stimulation for fertility preservation or family building in a cohort of transgender men. J Assist Reprod Genet. 2019;36:2155–61.

Al-Inany HG, Youssef MA, Ayeleke RO, Brown J, Lam WS, Broekmans FJ. Gonadotrophin-releasing hormone antagonists for assisted reproductive technology. Cochrane Database Syst Rev. 2016 Apr 29;4(4):CD001750.

Anderson RA, Amant F, et al. ESHRE Guideline Group on Female Fertility Preservation. ESHRE guideline: female fertility preservation. Hum Reprod Open. 2020 Nov 14;2020(4):hoaa052.

Armuand G, Dhejne C, Olofsson JI, Rodriguez-Wallberg KA. Transgender men's experiences of fertility preservation: a qualitative study. Hum Reprod. 2017;32:383–90.

Ata B, Capuzzo M, Turkgeldi E, Yildiz S, La Marca A. Progestins for pituitary suppression during ovarian stimulation for ART: a comprehensive and systematic review including meta-analyses. Hum Reprod Update. 2021 Jan 4;27(1):48–66.

Boots CE, Meister M, Cooper AR, Hardi A, Jungheim ES. Ovarian stimulation in the luteal phase: systematic review and meta-analysis. J Assist Reprod Genet. 2016;33:971–80.

Bosch E, Broer S, Griesinger G, Grynberg M, Humaidan P, Kolibianakis E, Kunicki M, La Marca A, Lainas G, et al. The ESHRE Guideline Group on Ovarian Stimulation, ESHRE guideline: ovarian stimulation for IVF/ICSI. Hum Reprod Open. 2020 May 1;2020(2):hoaa009.

Cavagna F, Pontes A, Cavagna M, Dzik A, Donadio NF, Portela R, Nagai MT, Gebrim LH. Specific protocols of controlled ovarian stimulation for oocyte cryopreservation in breast cancer patients. Curr Oncol. 2018;25:e527–32.

Chen C. Pregnancy after human oocyte cryopreservation. Lancet 1986;1: 884–6.

Cobo A, Coello A, de los Santos MJ, Giles J, Pellicer A, Remohi J, García-Velasco JA. Number needed to freeze: cumulative live birth rate after fertility preservation in women with endometriosis. Reprod Biomed Online. 2021;42:725–32.

Cobo A, García-Velasco J, Domingo J, Pellicer A, Remohí J. Elective and onco-fertility preservation: factors related to IVF outcomes. Hum Reprod. 2018 Dec 1;33(12):2222–31.

Cobo A, Giles J, Paolelli S, Pellicer A, Remohi J, Garcia-Velasco JA. Oocyte vitrification for fertility preservation in women with endometriosis: an observational study. Fertil Steril. 2020;113:836–44.

Dondorp W, de Wert G, Pennings G, Shenfield F, Devroey P, Tarlatzis B, et al. Oocyte cryopreservation for age-related fertility loss. Human Reprod. 2012 May;27(5):1231–7.

Glujovsky D, Pesce R, Sueldo C, Quinteiro Retamar AM, Hart RJ, Ciapponi A. Endometrial preparation for women undergoing embryo transfer with frozen embryos or embryos derived from donor oocytes. Cochrane Database Syst Rev. 2020 Oct 28;10(10):CD006359.

Kuang Y, Chen Q, Fu Y, Wang Y, Hong Q, Lyu Q, et al. Medroxyprogesterone acetate is an effective oral alternative for preventing premature luteinizing hormone surges in women undergoing controlled ovarian hyperstimulation for in vitro fertilization. Fertil Steril. 2015;104(1):62–70.

Kuang Y, Chen Q, Hong Q, Lyu Q, Ai A, Fu Y, Shoham Z. Double stimulations during the follicular and luteal phases of poor responders in IVF/ICSI programmes (Shanghai protocol). Reprod Biomed Online. 2014;29:684–91.

Labarta E, Mariani G, Paolelli S, Rodriguez-Varela C, Vidal C, Giles J, Bellver J, Cruz F, Marzal A, Celada P, Olmo I, Alamá P, Remohi J, Bosch E. Impact of low serum progesterone levels on the day of embryo transfer on pregnancy outcome: a prospective cohort study in artificial cycles with vaginal progesterone. Hum Reprod. 2021 Feb 18;36(3):683–692.

Leung A, Sakkas D, Pang S, Thornton K, Resetkova N. Assisted reproductive technology outcomes in female-to-male transgender patients compared with cisgender patients: a new frontier in reproductive medicine. Fertil Steril. 2019;112:858–65.

Marklund A. Efficacy and safety of controlled ovarian stimulation using GnRH antagonist protocols for emergency fertility preservation in young women with breast cancer — a prospective nationwide Swedish multicenter study. Hum Reprod. 2020 Apr 28;35(4):929–38.

Mathieu d'Argent E, Ferrier C, Zacharopoulou C, Ahdad-Yata N, Boudy AS, Cantalloube A, Levy R, Antoine JM, Daraï E, Bendifallah S. Outcomes of fertility preservation in women with endometriosis: comparison of progestin-primed ovarian stimulation versus antagonist protocols. J Ovarian Res. 2020 Feb 13;13(1):18.

Mumusoglu S, Polat M, Ozbek IY, Bozdag G, Papanikolaou EG, Esteves SC, Humaidan P, Yarali H. Preparation of the endometrium for frozen embryo transfer: a systematic review. Front Endocrinol (Lausanne). 2021 Jul 9;12:688237.

Oktay K, Turkcuoglu I, Rodriguez-Wallberg KA. GnRH agonist trigger for women with breast cancer undergoing fertility preservation by aromatase inhibitor/FSH stimulation. Reprod Biomed Online. 2010;20:783–8.

Practice Committees of the American Society for Reproductive Medicine and the Society for Assisted Reproductive Technology. Mature oocyte cryopreservation: a guideline. Fertil Steril. 2013;99:37–43.

Rodgers RJ, Reid GD, Koch J, Deans R, Ledger WL, Friedlander M, Gilchrist RB, Walters KA, Abbott JA. The safety and efficacy of controlled ovarian hyperstimulation for fertility preservation in women with early breast cancer: a systematic review. Hum Reprod. 2017;32:1033–45.

Vaiarelli A, Cimadomo D, Trabucco E, Vallefuoco R, Buffo L, Dusi L, Fiorini F, Barnocchi N, Bulletti FM, Rienzi L, et al. Double stimulation in the same ovarian cycle (DuoStim) to maximize the number of oocytes retrieved from poor prognosis patients: A multicenter experience and SWOT analysis. Front Endocrinol (Lausanne). 2018;9:317.

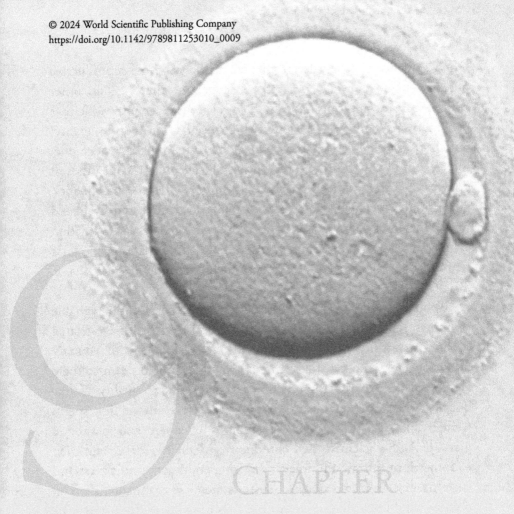

CHAPTER

The Application of Artificial Intelligence to Oocyte Evaluation:
Methods, Scope and Limitations

Rachel Smith and Dan Nayot

Oocyte quality is an elusive term used to describe the reproductive potential of an oocyte. Other than female age, there are no other clinical features that can predictably correlate with fecundity. Neither imaging nor bloodwork provides further insights into oocyte quality; rather, ovarian reserve markers, such as anti-Müllerian hormone, follicle-stimulating hormone and antral follicle count, are measures of oocyte quantity, and are essentially independent from quality. Surprisingly, even when oocytes are finally extracted and evaluated under the light microscope, there is no validated visual evaluation system that provides clinically meaningful information on their reproductive potential (Alpha Scientists in Reproductive Medicine, 2012).

By all measures, a viable oocyte is usually the rate-limiting variable in human reproduction. This is clearly demonstrated with age-related decline in fertility which can generally be overcome with younger donor oocytes. And yet, for such a critical and limited resource there are no established evaluation methods to determine its quality. Unlike oocytes, there are established visual evaluation criteria for sperm (semen analysis; WHO, 2021), embryos (cleavage and blastocyst grading; Alpha Scientists in Reproductive Medicine, 2012) and even endometrium (ultrasound images assessing endometrial thickness and pattern). If a validated oocyte scoring system was available, then all oocytes would be subjected to it regardless of whether they were to be discarded, donated, cryopreserved or inseminated to generate an embryo.

Embryologists currently assess the oocytes by rudimentary means. Initial oocyte assessments focus on the cumulus-oocyte complex, ideally observing an expanded cumulus, often referred to as cloud-like, with a radiating corona (Alpha Scientists in Reproductive Medicine, 2012), which can be indicative of nuclear maturity. If oocytes are to be cryopreserved, or inseminated via intracytoplasmic sperm injection (ICSI), then the cumulus cells are denuded ("stripped"). At this stage nuclear maturity can be clearly identified and classified as germinal vesicle, metaphase I or metaphase II (MII) respectively based on the presence or absence of both the geminal vesicle nucleus and first polar body. Assessing cytoplasmic maturity is much less concrete. Oocyte morphology commentary focuses on both cytoplasmic (granularity, clusters, vacuoles, inclusions, etc.) and extra-cytoplasmic (zona pellucida, perivitelline space and polar body) features.

Although a systematic review highlighted that no specific morphological features were unanimously evaluated to have prognostic value for further developmental competence of oocytes (Rienzi et al, 2011), there remains a common belief that the lack of dysmorphisms represents a high-quality oocyte. For features suggestive of sub-optimal quality see Figures 9.1 and 9.2. The Istanbul Consensus Workshop 2011 defined an optimal mature oocyte morphology as a spherical

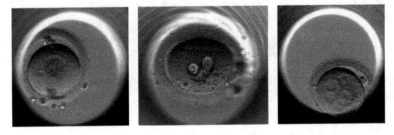

Figure 9.1   Cytoplasmic dysmorphisms: (from left) central granulation, multiple vacuoles, multiple smooth endoplasmic reticula.

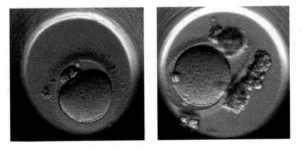

Figure 9.2   Extra-cytoplasmic features: (from left) large polar body, irregular zona pellucida.

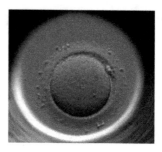

Figure 9.3 Mature oocyte (MII) that would be assumed to be of high quality.

structure enclosed by a uniform zona pellucida, with a uniform translucent cytoplasm free of inclusions and a size-appropriate polar body (Figure 9.3).

A classic example on the limitations of relying on oocyte dysmorphisms as a measure of oocyte quality is the presence of smooth endoplasmic reticula (sER) within the cytoplasm. Some earlier studies reported that the sER oocytes had lower *in vitro* fertilisation (IVF) success rates, as well as increased obstetrical complications and neonatal outcomes. This led to the common practice of discarding sER oocytes altogether to minimise the risk of any downstream harm. More recent studies have questioned the degree of these reported negative outcomes from sER oocytes, if any at all. Currently many IVF labs either deselect sER oocytes to their last-priority embryo (if it had led to a blastocyst) or ignore it as a prognostic variable.

A successful IVF cycle requires a viable embryo be transferred to a receptive endometrium. Unfortunately, even as our field continues to evolve, most IVF cycles are still unsuccessful, and both patients and clinicians are seeking insights into the aetiology or at least the limiting factor to account for the failed treatment cycle. Embryo quality is a downstream result of both sperm and oocyte quality. Information about sperm quality is inferred by the semen analysis of the sample and post-processing analytics, but insights into oocyte quality remain vague and are generally based on female age and subsequent embryology outcomes.

The lack of information on oocyte quality is magnified in oocyte cryopreservation cases, where subsequent embryo development is not available to provide immediate, but indirect, feedback on those oocytes. Oocyte cryopreservation is now common practice around the world for fertility preservation, oocyte donation, and in some countries is part of routine practice due to legislative or religious restrictions requiring limitations in creating supernumerary embryos.

Specifically in oocyte cryopreservation, predictions about live birth success rates are based on historical modelling considering only two key variables: female age at the time of oocyte extraction and the number of mature oocytes cryopreserved. This of course is an over-simplification assuming that all oocytes in the cohort have the same average potential and that oocyte quality is strictly defined by female age. This general feedback to patients is considered the standard of care in oocyte cryopreservation cases until an oocyte quality assessment tool becomes available.

Having an effective method to evaluate oocytes so as to inform patients of oocyte quality allows for improved decision making, empowers patient choices, and may maximise the chance of a successful outcome.

A universal oocyte grading system would also benefit inter-laboratory comparisons, quality assurance and laboratory key performance indicators, driving standards to improve oocyte quality.

9.1 Other Oocyte Evaluation Methods

Visual: As highlighted, embryologists can visually identify and comment on several aspects of the oocytes using a standard light microscope, but oocyte dysmorphisms do not consistently correlate with the reproductive potential of oocytes. If in fact dysmorphisms were known to be negative or positive predictors of blastocyst development or ploidy status, then an oocyte scoring system could easily be generated by combining individual dysmorphisms as an aggregated score.

Other attempts to visually evaluate oocytes include using polarised microscopy to assess the polar body presence, positioning and birefringence (Oosight® by Hamilton Thorne). Intracellular temperature imaging has also been investigated as an objective tool to assess oocyte competence, as the intracellular temperature and temperature distribution differ between oocytes and could be an indicator of oocyte quality once phenomena within the cell are mapped definitively (Hoshino, 2018).

Non-Visual: There are non-visual approaches to gather more information about sperm (e.g., DNA fragmentation), embryos (e.g., preimplantation genetic testing for aneuploidy or PGT-A) and endometrium (e.g., endometrial biopsy assays). Similarly, there is ongoing research to evaluate oocytes by different means including mechanical pressure dynamics, cumulus cell bioanalysis (proteomic, metabolomics, etc.), and polar body biopsies.

Research into follicular fluid biomarkers linked to oocyte competence have been identified and showed promising results, but in practice utilising this technology is restrictive due to sampling challenges, traceability, time constraints and cost consideration (Sirait et al, 2021).

However, a validated visual oocyte scoring system to identify oocytes with higher or lower reproductive potential has yet to be developed.

9.2 The Application of Artificial Intelligence to Oocytes

This chapter will highlight how the emergence of artificial intelligence (AI) image analysis can tackle the 'black box' of oocyte quality. Trained embryologists rely on their experience, but they do not have an endless feedback loop to learn from the fate of each oocyte. Their dysmorphism "diagnosis" is inherently subjective with known inter- and intra-observer variability. Even the most experienced embryologists can only detect finite patterns in grey scale to a certain size limit, as opposed to computers that can process at the pixel level of images. There is a real need for a quantitative, detailed, consistent, non-invasive method of analysing the key factors to indicate oocyte competence.

AI is a rapidly evolving field and can be classified as software programs with the ability to learn and reason like humans. Machine learning (ML) is a subset of AI with algorithms that have the ability to learn without explicitly being programmed, and deep learning is a subset of machine learning in which artificial neural networks adapt and learn from vast amounts of data. The application of AI in healthcare is in its infancy but accelerating quickly in terms of clinical applications, functionality, and acceptance.

In theory, AI should be superior to embryologists in their ability to assess oocyte quality since even the most experienced embryologists are limited by their innate senses. Human vision is restricted by its ability to perceive and analyse, whereas applying AI to image analysis can identify features that are otherwise unrecognisable by embryologists. A clinically meaningful oocyte scoring system should correlate with the reproductive potential of that oocyte, whether within the IVF lab (from successful fertilisation to blastocyst development) or beyond the IVF lab (onto implantation, an established clinical pregnancy and, ultimately, a healthy live birth).

In reproductive medicine, AI has been applied to support clinical decision making (such as suggested treatment protocol or the ideal time to trigger ovulation) as well as to improve sperm and embryo selection. AI offers promise for the automation, standardisation and improved assessment of many applications, and is quickly gaining attention as an inevitable innovation within the IVF lab.

Some pillars for a successful AI application should include a defined clinical problem, a high quality and large data set, and appropriate validation studies.

There is no validated visual oocyte scoring system in clinical practice. Embryologists are unable to predict the reproductive potential of oocytes. Patients with cryopreserved oocytes have no insights into their oocyte quality and rely on general feedback based on female age and the number of mature oocytes frozen.

The development of an AI tool for oocyte assessment requires as inputs high-quality single two-dimensional images of denuded MII oocytes and as an output a defined primary outcome with binary labelling. An example of an ideal primary end point is a utilisable blastocyst, defined as a day 5 or 6 embryo suitable for biopsy (PGT-A) or cryopreservation for subsequent frozen embryo transfer.

To focus on the reproductive potential of the oocyte, it would be ideal to restrict the analysis to normal sperm samples (no male factor) such that poor outcomes (e.g., no fertilisation or embryo arrest) can be attributed to the oocyte's contribution.

Generally, the larger the data set the more accurate the AI algorithm can reach, although there is a natural limit where more data would not yield further benefits. Additionally, a more diverse data set (patient population, IVF lab conditions) will improve the robustness of the algorithm.

In all scientific studies, there is a hierarchy in study designs for validation. At the very least, any image prediction tool should run the AI algorithm on a test data set of images not previously seen by the program (blind set) in both an unbalanced and balanced sample (retrospective study). Clearly demonstrating that the AI program can outperform the current standard of care would be important. In the case of oocyte quality, this translates to comparing the predictive ability of the AI algorithm to a trained embryologist (as there is no standardised oocyte evaluation to serve as a baseline) in a test set. A reproducibility study with similar results in independent conditions (images of oocytes from another IVF lab) would strengthen the evidence. Finally, a prospective study in real-time conditions would be the next evolution of a validation study.

9.3 Oocyte Artificial Intelligence: Development of Violet™

The clinical goal was to develop an AI software program (named Violet™) to correlate between the image of a denuded MII and its chance of developing into a utilisable blastocyst, i.e., a visual oocyte quality tool (Figure 9.4). Any ability to predict the IVF embryological outcomes from analysing the mature oocyte would represent an improvement on the current standard of care, which is unable to do so. This technology can be applied to elective oocyte cryopreservation by providing personalised predictions on each oocyte or the full cohort. In oocyte donation programs such a technology can optimise a more balanced distribution between intended parents or assist in deciding the number of oocytes that should be frozen per batch to get a desired number of blastocyst outcomes.

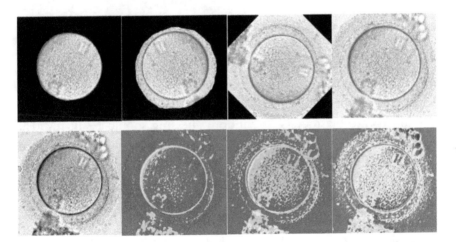

Figure 9.4 Examples of processed oocyte images used to train Violet™: (Top row, from left) scaled oocyte image, segmented image to the oolemma, segmented image to the perivitelline space, rotated oocyte. (Bottom row, from left) Oocyte with modified contrast and blurred oocyte, heat amp of contrast oocyte in three colour ways.

The original unbalanced data set included 15,013 data points (images of denuded MII oocytes and subsequent blastocyst development outcomes), of which 6,721 oocytes were labelled as blastocyst positive and 8,292 oocytes labelled as blastocyst negative (failed fertilisation, embryo arrest or embryos discarded due to poor-quality grading and determined to be not utilisable). The database was randomly split into three subsets as: Training, Validation and Testing, in ratios of 70%, 20%, and 10%, respectively.

In a retrospective, blinded and unbalanced data set Violet™ was able to predict blastocyst development with 62% accuracy, based on a single image. Violet™ was especially effective at identifying negative cases with 99% accuracy when the confidence was >70%. Performance of the unbalanced data set for blastocyst development received an area-under-curve score of 0.666 and mean recall score of 0.621 (recall negative score: 0.608, recall positive score: 0.634).

9.3.1 Artificial Intelligence vs Humans

A subset of 300 test images were set aside for testing the model against 17 senior embryologists from eight IVF clinics (Figure 9.5). The 300 oocyte images were balanced, meaning 50% of the oocytes had developed into blastocysts, so random guessing should result in 50% accuracy. Both embryologists and Violet™ were blinded to true outcomes of the oocytes and were not given any information about the patients. Embryologists were not given any time restrictions to evaluate the oocytes and were also asked to rank their confidence in their predictions.

Violet™ outperformed all 17 embryologists in accurately predicting blastocyst development (62.8% vs 52.1% ± 3.4% standard deviation; p-value < 0.001). The exercise took the embryologists an average of two hours to complete, and was essentially instantaneous for Violet™. The inability of embryologists to predict the oocytes' potential to reach a blastocyst was confirmed (52.1% accuracy). Interestingly, the

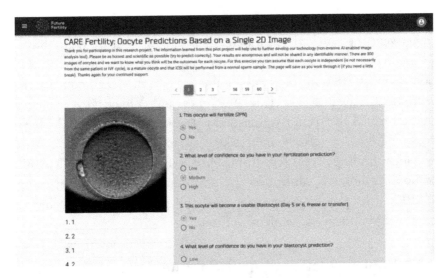

Figure 9.5   Oocyte predictions for embryologist evaluation.

embryologists' confidence in their prediction did not correlate with their accuracy. Violet™ had improved 20.5% in blastocyst prediction accuracy, compared to the embryologists.

A repeatability study was performed on the same task and images 2–3 months later by seven of the embryologists and Violet™. The average embryologist's accuracy remained close to chance, 54.0% ± 2.6% standard deviation (p-value < 0.001) with an intra-observer repeatability of 81.4% for blastocyst formation, while Violet™ was 100% repeatable.

The introduction of AI into the clinical setting takes careful consideration as most embryologists, doctors and patients have little background knowledge in the basics of AI or its limitations. Prior to the implementation it is advisable to validate the performance of the AI model on data derived from the local setting to ensure reproducible results are obtained from different conditions than those on which the model was derived.

CARE Fertility undertook a retrospective analysis providing 784 mature oocyte images — blinded for outcome for interpretation by

Violet™. Furthermore, 10 experienced embryologists at the clinic underwent the same AI vs Human challenge to compare their ability to predict fertilisation and blastocyst from a 2D static image of 300 oocytes taken from the original 784 images. The model outcomes were reproducible against the true outcomes and Violet™ once again outperformed all 10 embryologists for blastocyst prediction (62.1% vs mean 52.8%), a relative increased accuracy of 18%, in line with previous findings reported from Future Fertility of 20.5%. This in-house validation confirmed the performance of the model using CARE's strict protocols, ensuring staff and patient confidence in the technology prior to its implementation.

9.3.2 Implementation of Artificial Intelligence Technologies for Oocyte Assessment in the IVF Laboratory

Following in-house validation, the next consideration is for the safe implementation of the AI technology within the laboratory. Additional equipment may be required for installing AI technology. The Violet™ software requires consistent image resolution of at least 500×500 pixels and recommends the Basler (**acA3088-57uc**) camera fitted to an inverted microscope. The microscope must have a camera port and an appropriate C-mount lens adaptor for use with the make and model of the microscope and camera. The camera is linked via a USB port to a computer with the capacity to run the image capture software on Windows 10. Support with this process is offered by Future Fertility, the software manufacturers, with multiple videos and supporting documents for the correct installation and use.

As part of the process validation, it is critical to define the patients/clinical scenarios that will benefit from the oocyte prediction technology; the possible impact on the laboratory workflow; whether this incurs an increase in treatment cost; alongside the communication and delivery of information to patients relating to their outcomes and collective decision making by the clinical and embryology teams.

As data sets increase, and AI technology advances, we anticipate the accuracy and robustness of an image analysis oocyte assessment tool to improve. There are other approaches to consider to extend its predictive potential, including adding important clinical variables (e.g., anti-Müllerian hormone levels, smoking status, etc.) and evaluating the oocyte in new approaches (e.g., multiple images from multiple angles). Similarly, the primary outcome will continue to evolve from a utilisable blastocyst, to a high-quality or PGT-A screened euploid blastocyst, or beyond including implantation and clinical pregnancy.

An oocyte AI tool solves a real clinical limitation for elective oocyte cryopreservation, but it can have a role in egg donor and ICSI cases as well. For egg donors, it can be used as a quality measure, as it is clear not all oocyte cohorts from young donors are of high quality. It can assist with lab-driven decision making like personalising the lot size for each donor case based on the intended outcome parameters (e.g., you may require nine oocytes from the current cohort to have a 75% chance of generating three blastocysts). Similarly, it could assist in fairly distributing the oocyte cohort among two or more intended parents to increase the chance of a balanced outcome for each recipient.

In ICSI cases, it might be used for oocyte selection in jurisdictions that restrict the number of oocytes that can be fertilised at once. Furthermore, it is logical to believe that using an oocyte assessment tool as part of your embryo selection criteria could improve outcomes.

9.4 Conclusion

Analogous to sperm, embryo and endometrium, a visual evaluation system for oocytes is needed in reproductive medicine and, if available, would be used routinely whenever oocytes are handled, i.e., oocyte freezing, oocyte donation, or oocyte usage in IVF-ICSI cycles.

Currently there is no validated oocyte scoring system, and a high-quality oocyte can only be commented on retrospectively based on its downstream reproductive success. For elective oocyte cryopreservation and oocyte donation cycles, the lack of insights into oocyte quality beyond nuclear maturity is evident in daily practice by the absence of a quantitative or semi-quantitative measure of oocyte competence. To create an oocyte evaluation system the oocyte quality assessment needs to correlate with the reproductive outcomes, such as blastocyst development. Unfortunately, it is currently not possible to predict the outcomes of oocytes just by visual evaluation, even by trained embryologists. The application of machine learning via analysis of two-dimensional images of mature denuded oocytes can shed valuable insights into oocyte quality. AI can additionally identify features that are otherwise unrecognisable by humans.

As with all AI image analysis tools, a larger and more diverse data set is necessary to extrapolate findings and a prospective multi-centre validation study should be strived for. The technology to accurately predict the reproductive potential of oocytes based on two-dimensional image analysis will continue to improve as data sets increase and deep learning techniques advance.

References

Alpha Scientists in Reproductive Medicine. The Alpha consensus meeting on cryopreservation key performance indicators and benchmarks: Proceedings of an expert meeting. Reprod Biomed Online. 2012 Aug;25(2):146–67.

Hoshino Y. Updating the markers for oocyte quality evaluation: Intracellular temperature as a new index. Reprod Med Biol. 2018 Sep 27;17(4): 434–41.

Rienzi L, Vajta G, Ubaldi F. Predictive value of oocyte morphology in human IVF: As systematic review of the literature. Hum Reprod Update. 2011 Jan–Feb;17(1):34–45.

Sirait B, Wiweko B, Jusuf AA, Iftitah D, Muharam R. Oocyte competence biomarkers associated with oocyte maturation: a review. Front Cell Dev Biol. 2021 Aug 30;9:710292.

WHO Laboratory manual for the examination and processing of human sperm, sixth edition. July 2021. https://www.who.int/publications/i/item/9789240030787

https://doi.org/10.1142/9789811253010_0010

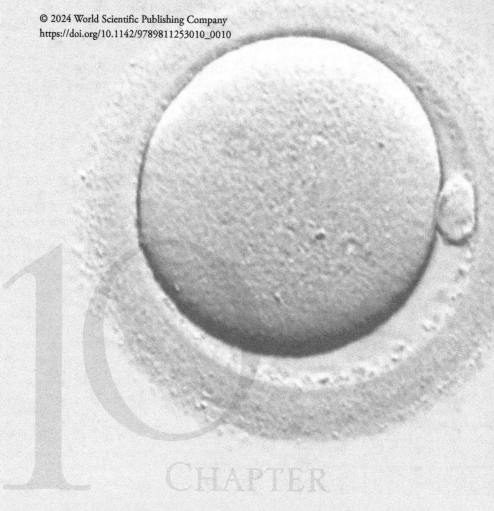

CHAPTER

Public Perceptions and Societal Attitudes versus Egg Freezing Realities

Marcia C. Inhorn and Pasquale Patrizio

10.1 Introduction

To understand public perceptions of egg freezing, it is necessary to begin with the announcement on 19 October 2012 by the American Society for Reproductive Medicine (ASRM) that the experimental label on oocyte vitrification was being lifted. Opening the door to egg freezing among otherwise healthy women, the ASRM still urged caution, pointing out that there were insufficient data on safety, success rates, cost effectiveness, and physical and emotional risks. Furthermore, reliable data on the ultimate success of egg freezing were not readily available. Thus, the viability of egg freezing and what it would ultimately mean for women and their future children remained highly uncertain. Having said this, the European Society for Human Reproduction and Embryology soon followed suit, lifting experimental restrictions by 2013.

In the United States, the focus of this chapter, many *in vitro* fertilisation (IVF) clinics began offering egg freezing cycles almost immediately, and some clinics also began creating their own frozen donor egg banking programs. Approximately 5,000 elective egg freezing cycles were undertaken in the US in 2013, the first full year of clinical approval (Ethics Committee, 2013). By the end of the decade, five times as many egg freezing cycles had been performed, signalling the significant demand for this new reproductive technology among American women. Furthermore, an important update in 2018 by the ASRM Ethics Committee deemed egg freezing to be a form of "planned oocyte cryopreservation for women seeking to preserve reproductive potential". ASRM deemed egg freezing an "emerging but ethically permissible procedure that may help women avoid future infertility" (Ethics Committee, 2018, p. 1022). But an important caveat stated that "because egg freezing is new and evolving, it is essential that women who are considering using it be informed about the uncertainties regarding its efficacy and long-term effects" (Ethics Committee, 2018, p. 1022).

10.2 Public Perceptions of Egg Freezing

ASRM's somewhat ambivalent stance — namely, technological optimism tinged with uncertainty — was echoed in the media portrayals of egg freezing over the same time period. As soon as egg freezing's experimental label was lifted in 2012, hundreds of news stories and opinion pieces began to be published, often emanating in the American media, then circulating rapidly around the globe. For example, egg freezing was almost immediately deemed a form of "fertility insurance", and a way for thirty-something women to "rewind the biological clock". With egg freezing, younger women in their twenties could potentially put their fertility "on hold" — "deferring", "delaying", and "postponing" their childbearing until their educations were completed and their careers established. The ability to "freeze fertility in time" — putting off childbearing until a later date, but still being able to use one's own younger and healthier eggs — was immediately heralded as a "reproductive revolution", equivalent to the 1960s' introduction of the birth control pill.

The New York Times was at the forefront of this egg freezing coverage. Fully six months before egg freezing's experimental label was lifted, *The New York Times* published its first cover story, one that focused on the potential benefits of egg freezing for would-be grandparents, who might "nudge" their thirty-something daughters by paying for egg freezing, thereby increasing their own chances for future grandchildren (Gootman, 2012). The second *New York Times* piece, published five days after egg freezing's experimental label was lifted, was an editorial written by health and science journalist Sarah Elizabeth Richards (2012). An early advocate of egg freezing, Richards told women readers, "We Need to Talk About Our Eggs." The following year, she published a book called *Motherhood, Rescheduled: The New Frontier of Egg Freezing and the Women Who Tried It*, based on her own and three other women's experiences of egg freezing undertaken during the experimental period (Richards, 2013).

However, the tone of *The New York Times'* coverage soon shifted. Stories increasingly focused on the problems of egg freezing, including unequal access to this costly procedure, uncertainties in egg survival rates after freezing and rewarming processes, lack of success among those who had attempted to use their frozen eggs, and the thousands of frozen eggs still remaining in storage, given that most women did not return to use them. *The New York Times* also began to question the promotion and financing of egg freezing. Stories focused on the "aggressive" marketing strategies directed toward younger millennial women by clinics that "really, really, really want to freeze your eggs" (La Ferla, 2018), luring them in through ethically questionable champagne-soaked egg freezing "parties" and incessant social media advertising (Caron, 2019; Patrizio et al, 2016). They also covered how egg freezing "benefits" from companies such as Facebook and Apple were actually conveying a "dark message" to women workers about the need for mandatory fertility postponement (Miller, 2014). Five out of six editorials on egg freezing published in the *The New York Times* between 2016 and 2020 were either negative or ambivalent in nature. Most were written by women who had undergone egg freezing with various painful and untoward outcomes.

One of the most powerful *New York Times* editorials published during this period pointed to egg freezing's discriminatory potential as an expensive technology for "White women only" (Allen, 2016). Indeed, stereotypical images of the kind of women who might turn to egg freezing were beginning to form in the media. First, these women were presumed to be White and economically privileged. Second, they were often referred to as "career women", a term, we must note, that has no masculine equivalent. Third, they were said to be "career driven", a term sometimes used in a pejorative sense to criticise women with ambitions. The implication was that freezing their eggs, either by choice or necessity, was presumably a way for these ambitious career women to climb the corporate ladder.

In short, over the first decade of egg freezing's existence, popular portrayals circulating widely in the media led to a host of dominant stereotypes about the kind of women who would freeze their eggs. These included: 1) *ambitious twenty-somethings,* planning for their future careers, while also taking time to date, party, and have fun; 2) *career-driven thirty-somethings,* climbing the corporate ladder so hard that they "forget to have children"; 3) *oppressed employees,* paid by firms to freeze their eggs and put off childbearing indefinitely for the sake of the corporation; and 4) *gullible victims,* lured into egg freezing through unethical practices and the egg freezing "party culture" of a profit-oriented fertility industry.

But were these stereotypes true? In a prescient article entitled "Portrayals of Healthy Women Seeking Oocyte Cryopreservation", bioethicist Heidi Mertes (2013) questioned whether these images of egg freezing women were, in fact, correct, or whether they oversimplified women's egg freezing motivations and experiences. Mertes pointed to the three distinct ways in which egg freezing women were being cast: first, as "selfish career-pursuing women"; second, as "victims of a male-oriented society that makes it difficult for women to combine motherhood with a good education or professional responsibilities"; and third, as "wise, proactive women who will not have to depend on oocyte donors should they suffer from age-related infertility" (Mertes, 2013, p. 141). But instead, Mertes asked: Might the absence of a male partner be the most common reason why otherwise healthy women are freezing their eggs?

10.3 Egg Freezing Stories

In this chapter, we attempt to answer Mertes' important question through an in-depth, ethnographic study conducted with more than a hundred American women who froze their eggs. These women were recruited through four American IVF clinics, two academic and two private, all located along the East Coast corridor or in the heart of

Silicon Valley in California. All of these IVF clinics had active egg freezing programs, some having participated in early clinical trials. In each clinic, we circulated a flyer seeking women volunteers for an interview-based study of those who had already undertaken the procedure.

Many of the women who volunteered were from our home state of Connecticut, especially from the cities of New Haven and Hartford, the state capital. However, over time, most of the women who joined the study came from other major American cities, including New York City, Baltimore, Maryland, Washington, DC, and the San Francisco Bay Area, including Silicon Valley. Reflecting the high degree of American professional mobility, many women had moved for their jobs. Thus, women also joined the study from Austin, Texas; Boston, Massachusetts; Chicago, Illinois; Denver, Colorado; Los Angeles, California; Savannah, Georgia; Seattle, Washington; St. Louis, Missouri; and the North Carolina "Research Triangle" cities of Raleigh, Durham, and Chapel Hill. Four women had relocated overseas for jobs in Europe, the Middle East, and Asia; thus, they participated across many time zones.

Given the potential sensitivity of this subject matter and the profound importance of research ethics, all of the women who volunteered were given an informed consent form to read and sign before agreeing to a confidential, audio-recorded interview in a private setting of their own choosing. No one refused to sign, and most women seemed eager to share their stories with the first author, a medical anthropologist with years of experience interviewing infertility and IVF patients. Conversations unfolded in a variety of quiet spaces, including women's homes and offices, libraries, cafés, restaurants, private rooms in IVF clinics, or the anthropologist's office at Yale University. Where it was not possible to meet because of distance, the interview was conducted online or by phone.

Conversations always began with a few basic demographic questions, asking each woman about her age, place of birth, residential history, education, employment, relationship status, and how she would describe her ethnicity and religion. Women were also asked a few key questions about reproductive history, including the age of menarche, contraceptive usage, and any reproductive problems experienced.

Each woman was then asked to tell her own egg freezing story, in her own words. Women were often eloquent and loquacious storytellers, describing their life circumstances at the time of egg freezing, the details of their decision-making process, and how their egg freezing procedures had unfolded. But women also spoke about their love lives, their relationships with family members, the support they received from friends, what they liked and did not like about their jobs, their experiences with online dating, their perceptions of men, and their opinions about reproductive healthcare in America. Women sometimes highlighted dimensions of their lives that are rarely covered in the egg freezing media, such as how religion affected perceptions of egg freezing's morality, or how egg freezing might serve a healing function after illness, heartbreak, or trauma.

All in all, audio-recorded interviews were carried out with 114 healthy women who had completed at least one cycle of egg freezing — making this the largest ethnographic interview-based study of egg freezing ever undertaken. As our findings show, egg freezing involves a particular demographic of highly educated professional women. But they are *not* turning to egg freezing for the career reasons most often portrayed in the media. Instead, they face other challenges in achieving what we would call the *three P's — partnership, pregnancy, and parenting*. In the next section, we describe this egg freezing demographic, including their major challenge in becoming mothers.

10.4 The Egg Freezing Demographic

Our study shows that American women who freeze their eggs are defined by eight key features. These women are: (1) racially and ethnically diverse, (2) secular, (3) late thirty-something, (4) high-earning, (5) highly educated, (6) successful professionals, (7) who are heterosexual but single, and/or (8) facing ongoing partnership problems. All eight features do not apply to every single woman, but these characteristics are widely shared across this group, having major relevance for the ways in which women's egg freezing experiences unfold.

Racially and Ethnically Diverse. Women who freeze their eggs come from a variety of racial and ethnic backgrounds — backgrounds that are reflective of the cosmopolitan urban areas in which professional women tend to live and where IVF clinics are also located. In this study, slightly more than two-thirds of women (69 percent) self-identified as White, but nearly one-third (31 percent) self-identified as non-White. Among these, Asian American women of East, Southeast, and South Asian heritage backgrounds comprised the single largest minority group, at 18 percent overall. Black, Latinx, and mixed-race women were also represented, comprising about 3 to 4 percent each of the study population. Women of Middle Eastern heritage, both Arab and Persian, also volunteered for the study at 2 percent of the total. Such minority participation in egg freezing has not been well represented in the American media. But suffice it to say here that egg freezing in the US is *not* limited to White women only.

Secular. Women of many religious backgrounds are also freezing their eggs, often with the explicit support of religious authorities (Inhorn et al, 2020). More than half of the women in this study (58 percent) had been raised in Christian households, almost evenly split between Protestants and Catholics. But the single largest group, nearly one-third of all women in the study, had been raised Roman Catholic. Catholic women may have particular moral concerns regarding egg freezing, because the Catholic Church is singularly restrictive, disallowing all forms of reproductive technology.

In contrast, Jewish religious authorities have been exceptionally supportive of egg freezing. Not surprisingly then, Jewish women were significantly overrepresented in the study at 18 percent of the total, even though Jews make up only 2.2 percent of the US population. Hindu and Muslim women, mostly from South Asian immigrant families, each made up 3 to 4 percent of the overall group, while women who identified as Buddhists comprised 2 percent of the total. Nearly 16 percent of women had no religious background, especially women from East Asian immigrant families, who often identified themselves as agnostic, atheist, or secular.

No matter their religious upbringing, 90 percent of egg freezing women said that they no longer practiced any kind of religion and considered themselves to be secular. Many women identified themselves as "spiritual but non-religious", a category that is growing among a younger generation of Americans (Pew Research Center, 2014).

Late Thirty-Something. As qualitative studies from around the world consistently show, women who freeze their eggs are in their late thirties, generally between the ages of 36 and 38 (e.g., see Baldwin, 2019 for the UK and Hammarberg et al, 2017 for Australia). This proved to be true in our study as well, where the average age at first egg freezing was 36.6. In fact, fully three-quarters (73 percent) of women in the study were in their late thirties (ages 35 to 39) by the time they chose egg freezing, and 10 percent were in their forties (ages 40 to 43). With more than four-fifths of women aged 35 and above, only 17 percent of women froze their eggs in their early thirties (ages of 30 to 34), indicating the degree to which egg freezing is a *late* thirty-something endeavour.

Only one woman was younger than 30 when she froze her eggs. But she was a special case, because her father was a retiring IVF physician who encouraged her to freeze her eggs before he left his practice. The stark absence of "twenty-somethings" in this and other egg freezing studies suggests that younger women have not yet been convinced to try this costly and invasive technology, including as a tool for career planning. Furthermore, cost-benefit analyses suggest that egg freezing does not really make sense for fertile twenty-somethings, many of whom will eventually partner and conceive without any technological assistance (Ben-Rafael, 2018). Instead, egg freezing is most applicable to the lives of thirty-something women, who are weighing the benefits of this technology against its high costs.

High-Earning. Indeed, egg freezing is expensive, averaging between $10,000 and $16,000 per cycle in the US, but costing anywhere from $7,500 to $18,000 per cycle, depending upon the IVF clinic and the amount and cost of accompanying medications. Women must also pay annual storage fees, which average between $500 and $1,000, but can range from $300 to $1,500, depending upon the clinic and its egg bank. If they return to use their frozen eggs, then they must pay for the second half of an IVF cycle, which includes rewarming the frozen eggs, fertilising them through intracytoplasmic sperm injection, and transferring the best quality embryo(s) to a woman's womb — a process that can cost an average of $6,000 additional dollars. Given these high costs, only women with substantial financial means can afford this technology, making it out of reach for the vast majority of American women.

In this study, most women were entirely self-supporting, and able to pay for egg freezing on their own. Although well-to-do parents often volunteered to pay for egg freezing cycles, nearly 90 percent of women were able to pay for their egg freezing cycles by themselves, relying on their salaries, savings accounts, family inheritances, or health insurance provided by their employers. More than half (57 percent) of the women had undertaken one egg freezing cycle, while one-third (31 percent) had undertaken two cycles, and 12 percent had undertaken three or four cycles, effectively multiplying their expenses.

Although women were not routinely asked about their salaries, a few reported high incomes in the six-figure range, for example,

$120,000, $148,000, $175,000, $200,000, $275,000, $325,000, $500,000, and $600,000. Such salaries put these women significantly above the $82,535 annual salary made by the average American taxpayer. Most of these egg freezing women were in the top 10 percent of earners (who average $158,002 annually), and some were in the top 5 percent (who average $309,348) (Kagan, 2021).

In short, most of these high-earning women could easily afford their egg freezing cycles. Still, their major recommendation was that the price be brought down to make the technology much more accessible and affordable to lower- and middle-income women, including some of their own friends and relatives. In our study, about 10 percent of women fell into this middle-income bracket. Even though most were well employed and self-supporting, they did not make such large salaries (for example, $70,000 as opposed to $170,000), and some were paying off substantial student loans. These women often struggled to put together the money for even one cycle, resorting to zero-interest credit cards, small loans, or depletion of their savings accounts. For example, a woman who worked as a federal regulator in a government agency in Washington, DC, had accumulated just enough money in her savings account to afford a $15,000 egg freezing cycle. But when only one egg was retrieved and frozen, she was bereft, considering her $15,000 expenditure to be "a sunk cost".

In contrast, an academic physician spent $35,000 from her savings on three cycles that produced 55 eggs, the highest number retrieved and frozen by any woman in this study. For her, egg freezing was inherently affordable, something that she compared to the cost of "another car". For most women, being able to afford these high-cost egg freezing cycles made the choice less difficult, and the egg freezing itself brought many women some measure of success and relief. Indeed, women in this study froze an average of 18 eggs — a number close to 20, which has been recommended for a woman in her late thirties to achieve at least one live birth (Goldman et al, 2017).

Highly Educated. Women's affluence was clearly tied to their high levels of education. Women in this study had not only completed university, nearly 80 percent of them had earned advanced degrees, including Master's degrees (45 percent), medical degrees (14 percent), doctoral degrees (10 percent), and law degrees (7 percent). More than 10 percent of all women had earned dual advanced degrees, such as MD-PhDs, MD-MPHs, and PhD-MPPs.

Furthermore, among these highly educated American women, one-third (32 percent) had attended Ivy League institutions, and another one-quarter (26 percent) had attended highly ranked public (e.g., the University of California-Berkeley) or private (e.g., Massachusetts Institute of Technology) universities. In other words, well over half (58 percent) of these American women had attended so-called "elite" academic institutions. As a group, they were exceptionally well-educated high achievers, whose years of schooling had prepared them for diverse and rewarding careers.

Successful Professionals. Most women in this study were not only gainfully employed, they were successful professionals with impressive job skills and sometimes remarkable career trajectories. Although women's job descriptions varied considerably, their careers tended to cluster in ten key areas. The largest single category consisted of (1) women in *healthcare*, including many physicians who had frozen their eggs, as well as nurses, nurse-practitioners, healthcare management professionals, and women in the pharmaceutical sector. The healthcare category was followed, in rank order, by (2) women in *government*, including many women who worked in federal agencies, in US scientific and medical organisations, on Capitol Hill, in the foreign service, or in the US military or intelligence; (3) women in *tech*, including women who had started or owned tech companies, or worked as engineers, designers, programmers, and finance directors in the IT industry; (4) women in *consultancies*, including women who worked as management consultants, political consultants, policy advisors, and lobbyists; (5) women in *communications,* including journalists, filmmakers, marketing and communications directors; (6) women in *business,* including women who worked for major corporations, as well as small business owners and entrepreneurs; (7) women in *law,* including public and private attorneys and those working in the legal profession in a variety of capacities; (8) women in the *arts,* including musicians, performers, actors, artists, and architects; (9) women in *psychology,* including clinical psychologists, licensed clinical social workers, and other types of therapists; and (10) women in *academia,* including university professors, graduate students, and private school teachers.

Because these women were in their late thirties, the vast majority were already well established in their careers, with the exception of a few graduate students and physicians still in training. Most women stressed that their careers had kept them busy, sometimes impinging upon their free time and energy for dating. But most women had always hoped to meet a partner along the way. Thus, they were not using egg freezing as a career planning strategy, nor as a way to further postpone their fertility for the sake of their professions.

Only one woman in the entire study had explicitly undertaken egg freezing for career advancement purposes. At age 30, she was significantly younger than most other women interviewed, had attended two Ivy League universities on the way to an advanced degree, and was using egg freezing en route to becoming a tech entrepreneur in Silicon Valley. She was clear that she needed to delay childbearing for at least a decade to accomplish her professional goals. She was also one of only three women who identified as bisexual. Thus, her profile was significantly different from the rest of the women in the study. Another one of the younger women, age 33, was less explicit about her intended fertility postponement. But she had just passed the difficult Foreign Service exam and had frozen her eggs in order to pursue her new career in Latin America.

In fact, deployment overseas was one of the only career paths that directly impinged upon women's lives in ways that led them to egg freezing. Ten percent of women in this study worked in "deployable" positions in humanitarian organisations, US foreign aid agencies, US diplomatic security, the US Foreign Service, and the US military. As they explained, they often faced long-term deployments overseas, sometimes lasting up to three years, with movement from one foreign country to another. Although they were not freezing their eggs for career advancement, their careers involved substantial personal sacrifices and a high degree of mobility, which made relationship formation very difficult and egg freezing seem necessary. Not surprisingly, all of these women were single, with only one having ever been married.

Four of these women were high-ranking, active-duty military officers and intelligence analysts, who had been deployed multiple times to war zones or "other dodgy places", as one of them put it. These women were all single and lamented the difficulties of finding a partner, given the dangers of their jobs, the military's anti-fraternisation policies, and the fact that most military men were already married. Additionally, freezing their eggs comforted these women and their families, lest their lives be lost in the line of duty. Recognising the dangers and sacrifices that military women must make, the Department of Defense attempted in 2016 to forward a bill offering subsidised egg freezing services to all female soldiers prior to deployment in combat zones. But as of this writing, no Republicans in Congress have signed onto this legislation (Kime, 2019).

Heterosexual but Single. As with all of the military women, 82 percent of all women in the study were single, with no partner in sight. All but three of these single women were heterosexual, and even the three bisexual women declared an interest in partnering and parenting with men. Yet, the lack of a partner was a shared feature of women's lives, as it has been in every egg freezing study conducted to date.

Single women in this study were of two types: the never married and currently unpartnered, and the previously partnered but broken up. Fully half of all women (51 percent) fell into the first category.

Some of these women had had one or more serious relationships in the distant past, but those relationships had ended some time ago. Some women had never been in a serious relationship, for reasons that they could not quite understand. Many of these single women expressed regret and puzzlement over how they had "ended up" this way. But without a partner, these single women had turned to egg freezing to "buy time", while continuing to search for a partner with the hope of future marriage and motherhood.

The second group of single women, nearly one-third (31 percent) of the total, were turning to egg freezing in the aftermath of relationship breakups. These included both divorces (17 percent) and breakups from long-term relationships and engagements (14 percent). Suffice it to say here that these relationship traumas were often painful, leaving women quite bereft. In such cases, egg freezing provided a path to healing, as women attempted to repair their disrupted life courses.

Facing Ongoing Partnership Problems. Between the never-married singles and the women whose relationships had ended, fully four-fifths of women in this study (82 percent) were single. Being single — or what other studies describe as "lack of a partner" — was the main reason why these women had frozen their eggs. But even women *with* partners faced ongoing partnership problems. In this study, about one-fifth (18 percent) of women had a partner at the time of egg freezing, but half of these relationships were unstable. Several women had met "new boyfriends" around the time of egg freezing. But in these cases, it was very difficult for them to ascertain whether the relationship was going to last. In other cases, women found themselves in very unstable relationships with partners who were immature, unsupportive, unready to have children, or unfaithful. In these cases, it was very unclear whether relationships would survive. In both cases, egg freezing was being undertaken as a kind of backup plan, to see whether a relationship would develop or fall apart.

Among the nearly 10 percent of women who were in stable relationships, women were undertaking egg freezing while waiting for their partners to be "ready" to have children. Men who were "unready" cited various reasons for their delay, for example, completion of advanced degrees or professional training, significant career moves, or in some cases, because they were significantly younger than their female partners. In other cases, men simply did not feel prepared to become fathers, and were asking their female partners to wait. In summary then, fully 91 percent of women in this study were either single (82 percent) or in a tenuous relationship (9 percent) — the relationship problems that underlie the egg freezing phenomenon.

10.5 Conclusion

Ultimately, then, women who freeze their eggs are doing so to try to give themselves a remaining chance of biologically connected motherhood. They freeze their eggs not to delay parenthood, but rather to enable it at a time when they have met the right partner with whom to become pregnant and have children. Egg freezing, we argue, is their *new hope technology*, allowing women to imagine what life would be like with the three important P's of partnership, pregnancy, and parenting.

However, highly educated American women face a difficult challenge — one that has been called the "men as partners" problem in international reproductive health circles (Dudgeon and Inhorn, 2004; Wentzell and Inhorn, 2014). To wit, reproduction is inherently relational. It requires both men and women, or at least their sperm and their eggs, to come together in procreation. Ideally, it also involves men's and women's emotional investments in one another and in their children. But the lack of stable reproductive partners for many of America's most highly educated women represents a "men as partners" problem that needs to be recognised, called out, and confronted. For the women in our study, this problem is having significant and deleterious consequences for their reproductive lives, forcing them into a demoralising state of reproductive suspension.

These highly educated professional women are often trying their hardest to find compatible male partners, with whom they can build families. But they face three major challenges: First, men who are simply reluctant to partner with high-achieving women, leaving these women single for many years. Second, men who are unready for marriage and children, often leading to relationship demise. Third, men who exhibit bad behaviour, such as infidelity or ageism, often leading to relationship instability and rupture. Because of these heterosexual relationship problems, otherwise accomplished American women are pursuing egg freezing as a stop-gap measure in an effort to preserve a path to motherhood.

Understanding these relationship realities and ruptures among marriage- and motherhood-minded American professional women shows that egg freezing is *not* about their career planning. The notion that women are freezing their eggs to "lean in" to their careers is simply incorrect (Sandberg, 2013). By extension, ASRM's advocacy of the term "planned" is probably misdirected, given that it too closely associates egg freezing with career planning, thereby overemphasising women's intentionality in this regard.

As our study shows, egg freezing is rarely about *planned fertility postponement*, in the sense of women actively "deferring", "delaying", or "postponing" their fertility for the sake of their professions. Rather, egg freezing is about *unplanned fertility preservation* among women who are hoping to retain and extend their remaining reproductive potential until they can find a partner with whom to have children. The reality that few single women return to use their frozen eggs is clear proof that egg freezing is not about planned fertility postponement. These single women have often waited years for a partner who never materialised, and most do not return for their frozen eggs in an attempt to become so-called "single mothers by choice" (Hertz, 2008).

In conclusion then, women's increasing turn to egg freezing has not arisen out of nowhere. In the US, the UK, and a growing number of societies where studies have been conducted, egg freezing represents a technological concession to the challenges women face in their attempts to form meaningful and lasting heterosexual relationships. Most American women who freeze their eggs wish that they could have children *now* in a committed relationship with a man they love. But in the absence of a partner, women are using egg freezing to preserve and extend their fertility, while hoping for a rare "unicorn" — namely, a man who wants an age-appropriate, equal relationship with a woman, and who is also interested in marriage and children — to sweep them off their feet.

References

Allen R. Is egg freezing only for white women? [Internet]. The New York Times; 2016 May 21. Available from: https://www.nytimes.com/2016/05/22/opinion/is-egg-freezing-only-for-white-women.html.

Baldwin K. Egg freezing, fertility and reproductive choice: Negotiating responsibility, hope and modern motherhood. Emerald Publishing; 2019.

Caron C. Wait, is that another ad for egg freezing? [Internet]. The New York Times; 2019 April 27. Available from: https://www.nytimes.com/2019/04/27/parenting/freezing-your-eggs-ads.html.

Dudgeon MR, Inhorn MC. Men's influences on women's reproductive health: Medical anthropological perspectives. Soc Sci Med. 2004 Oct; 59(7):1379–95.

Ethics Committee of the American Society for Reproductive Medicine. Oocyte or embryo donation to women of advanced age: A committee opinion. Fertil Steril. 2013 Aug;100(2):337–40.

Ethics Committee of the American Society for Reproductive Medicine. Planned oocyte cryopreservation for women seeking to preserve future reproductive potential: an Ethics Committee opinion. Fertil Steril. 2018 Nov;110(6):1022–28.

Goldman RH, Racowsky C, Farland LV, Munné S, Ribustello L, Fox JH. Predicting the likelihood of live birth for elective oocyte cryopreservation: A counseling tool for physicians and patients. Hum Reprod. 2017 Apr 1; 32(4):853–59.

Gootman E. So eager for grandchildren, they're paying the egg-freezing clinic [Internet]. The New York Times; 2012 May 14. Available from: https://www.nytimes.com/2012/05/14/us/eager-for-grandchildren-and-putting-daughters-eggs-in-freezer.html.

Hammarberg K, Kirkman M, Pritchard N, Hickey M, Peate M, McBain J, Agresta F, Bayly C, Fisher J. Reproductive experiences of women who cryopreserved oocytes for non-medical reasons. Hum Reprod. 2017 Mar 1; 32(3):575–81.

Hertz R. Single by chance, mothers by choice: how women are choosing parenthood without marriage and creating the new American family. Oxford University Press; 2008.

Inhorn MC, Birenbaum-Carmeli D, Vale MD, Patrizio P. Abrahamic traditions and egg freezing: religious women's experiences in local moral worlds. Soc Sci Med. 2020 May;253:112976.

Kagan J. How much income puts you in the top 1%, 5%, 10%? [Internet]. Investopedia; 2021 June 10. Available from: https://www.investopedia.com/personal-finance/how-much-income-puts-you-top-1-5-10/.

Kime P. Bill would require DoD to pay for combat troops to freeze sperm, eggs [Internet]. Military.com; 2019 March 19. Available from: https://www.military.com/daily-news/2019/03/19/bill-would-require-dod-pay-combat-troops-freeze-sperm-eggs.html.

La Ferla R. These companies really, really, really want to freeze your eggs [Internet]. The New York Times; 2018 August 29. Available from: https://www.nytimes.com/2018/08/29/style/egg-freezing-fertility-millennials.html.

Mertes H. The portrayal of healthy women requesting oocyte cryo-preservation. Facts Views Vis Obgyn. 2013;5(2):141–6.

Miller CC. Freezing eggs as part of employee benefits: some women see darker message [Internet]. The New York Times; 2014 October 14. Available from: https://www.nytimes.com/2014/10/15/upshot/egg-freezing-as-a-work-benefit-some-women-see-darker-message.html.

Patrizio P, Molinari E, Caplan A. Ethics of medical and nonmedical oocyte cryopreservation. Curr Opin Endocrinol Diabetes Obes. 2016 Dec;23(6):470–5.

Pew Research Center. The religious landscape study [Internet]. Pew Research Center; 2014. Available from: https://www.pewforum.org/religious-landscape-study/.

Richards SE. Motherhood rescheduled: the new frontier of egg freezing and the women who tried it. Simon & Schuster; 2013.

Richards SE. We need to talk about our eggs [Internet]. The New York Times; 2012 October 22. Available from: https://www.nytimes.com/2012/10/23/opinion/we-need-to-talk-about-our-eggs.html.

Sandberg S. Lean in: women, work, and the will to lead. Knopf; 2013.

Wentzell EA, Inhorn MC. Reconceiving masculinity and 'men as partners' for ICPD Beyond 2014: insights from a Mexican HPV study. Glob Public Health. 2014;9(6):691–705.

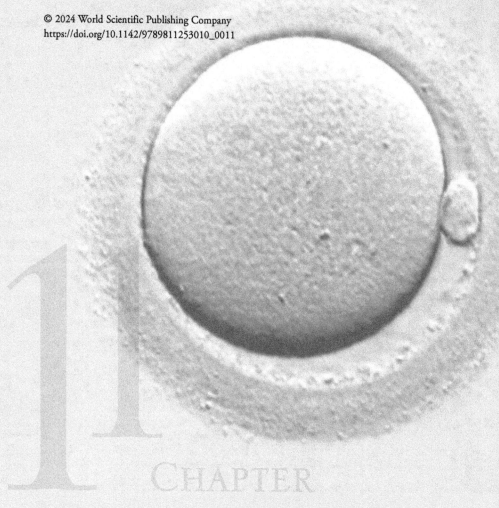

CHAPTER

Funding the Future
Family: An Unsettled Moral Issue

Molly Johnston and Michiel De Proost

11.1 Introduction

Interest in and demand for egg freezing is rapidly rising around the world (Cascante, 2023). Previously reserved for women facing premature infertility because of illness or medical treatments ('medical' egg freezing), egg freezing is now frequently used to help manage the threat of age-related fertility decline ('non-medical' egg freezing, also known as 'social', 'elective' or 'planned' egg freezing). In many nations there has been a shift in the timing of parenthood, with many individuals pursuing parenthood later in life (Beaujouan & Sobotka, 2022). While the reasons for this shift are likely to be multifaceted, freezing eggs at younger ages may help manage reproductive timelines against social and professional demands and preserve a chance of genetic parenthood (Inhorn, 2023).

Feature articles in the media often describe egg freezing as an imperative for modern women, for example using directive titles such as *"Egg Freezing Should be Every Dad's Graduation Present to Their Daughter"* and *"Egg Freezing: The Perfect 30th Birthday Gift for Women"*. An implicit question often embedded in these articles is who should pay for egg freezing and whether individuals (or their families) should cope privately with the financial burdens.

The cost of egg freezing is significant, ranging from US$7,500 to US$18,000 per cycle (Inhorn, 2023). The high costs have triggered academic and social debate regarding whether there is a societal obligation to aid individuals to access the procedure. The costs of egg freezing are frequently reported as a barrier to access, so there are calls for (greater) funding to reduce financial barriers. However, concerns have been raised about subsidising the costs, particularly regarding the option of publicly funding egg freezing, including whether it conveys the right moral message about parenthood.

Despite ongoing debate, some nations have introduced public funding for egg freezing but in varying degrees. In most instances the distinction between medical and non-medical egg freezing is used to determine access to funding. For example, in Australia, egg freezing on the grounds of a medical risk to fertility, such as illnesses or gonado-toxic treatments, is supported with a rebate through the public health system, Medicare. Approximately 50% of treatment costs are covered and there are no limits on the number of cycles eligible for rebate. However, non-medical egg freezing is not eligible to receive a rebate and the costs must be self-funded. Similar arrangements can be seen across Europe; a survey of European countries reported that of the 27 nations who responded, 14 offered some sort of funding, either through the public system or compulsory insurance, but only if egg freezing was medically indicated (Shenfield et al, 2017). Even among countries that provide funding, the structure that funding policies take differs. For example, in Denmark, funding covers the complete procedural and laboratory costs associated with medical egg freezing but coverage for medication is limited. Whereas in Ireland, only the costs of medication for treatment are publicly funded and the procedure itself must be self-funded (Calhaz-Jorge et al, 2020).

Until recently the use of the medical/non-medical distinction to determine eligibility for funding of egg freezing has not been challenged in public policy. However, in August of 2021, after multiple years of deliberation and debate, France's government enacted the new Bioethics Law. This law transforms and widens the provision of assisted reproductive technologies (ARTs) in France, where previously a more conservative regime had applied. What is particularly striking in the revised law is not only that France legalised non-medical egg freezing (previously, non-medical egg freezing was only permitted if a proportion of the eggs collected were donated), but that partial funding would be available to cover the associated procedural costs, making France the first jurisdiction in the world to publicly fund non-medical egg freezing. As we have argued elsewhere (De Proost and Johnston, 2021), this move challenges the justification for using the medical/non-medical distinction to determine access to funding.

These examples demonstrate the diversity between not just the approach taken to funding egg freezing in general, but also the structure that the policies take in nations where funding for egg freezing is available. There appears to be no consensus as to whether egg freezing should be publicly funded, nor how this should be done.

In this chapter we consider the different funding schemes for egg freezing. We will start by introducing the various schemes that have been made available through the private sector. These schemes have emerged to supposedly bridge the gap between high costs and access but, as we discuss, remain ethically ambiguous. We will then consider the question as to whether egg freezing should be publicly funded by critically evaluating some of the arguments made for and against. We conclude that unlike other ARTs, it is far from clear if, and if so how, funding for egg freezing should be offered within existing healthcare systems. Although public funding for egg freezing seems morally sound and intuitively correct within societies that already generously fund other ARTs, there may be good collective reasons to argue against the funding of egg freezing. Below, we consider alternative financing schemes.

11.2 Alternative Financing Schemes

11.2.1 Employer-sponsored Egg Freezing

In 2014 some Silicon Valley companies started offering to cover the costs of egg freezing for their female employees as an employee benefit. Apple, one of the first to implement the scheme, provides up to US$20,000 for employees interested in pursuing egg freezing. Since 2014, many other companies have followed suit, with some figures indicating that around one in five large (>20,000 employees) US companies now offer employer-sponsored egg freezing (Dowling, 2021). There has been significant academic and public debate regarding the expansion of employer-sponsored egg freezing (Johnston et al,

2022). Some have hailed it as a liberating move that expands reproductive options and promotes reproductive autonomy, while others have raised concerns that it disempowers women and confines reproductive autonomy, as women may feel pressured to freeze their eggs or risk not being considered competitive in the workforce. Although the literature is limited, women employed at companies that offer employer-sponsored egg freezing report not feeling pressured to freeze their eggs, but do acknowledge that employer-sponsored egg freezing does not resolve the challenges of navigating family planning and career development (Miner et al, 2020).

11.2.2 Freeze and Share

Not long after the experimental label was dropped from egg freezing in 2012, *Freeze and Share* egg share schemes were launched across the UK as well as in some other European nations. These schemes provide women with free access to egg freezing in exchange for donating a proportion (usually half) of their collected eggs to supply egg donor programs. It has been proposed that this scheme may work to overcome financial barriers for those who may wish to freeze their eggs, as well as providing a stream of donor eggs to relieve donor gamete shortages and assist others in conceiving.

There are certainly ethical concerns with this scheme. In particular, there is the validity of consent and risk of exploitation if there is a financial incentive to donate eggs, as well the potential emotional toll if the egg recipient's attempt to conceive is successful but the donor's future attempts are not. In addition, given that using frozen eggs to conceive is a two-step process, it is possible that despite being framed as an affordable option for those seeking egg freezing, *Freeze and Share* may not actually assist people to conceive, if those who received subsidised egg freezing cannot afford the future costs of thawing, fertilising and transferring the resulting embryos. Beyond the impact these schemes may have on those accessing them are broader questions around whether providing access to egg freezing is appropriate compensation for egg donation or whether it is more akin to an inducement (which should be rejected in jurisdictions that operate under an altruistic model of donation).

11.2.3 Egg Freezing-only Clinics

In 2016 the first egg freezing-only clinic was opened by the equity-backed company *Extend Fertility* in the US. Since the launch of *Extend Fertility* several other private egg freezing clinics have opened. Many of these private clinics employ various marketing tactics to attract patients, for example 'egg freezing parties', where egg freezing is discussed amongst cocktails and canapes, and sponsored advertisements through social media channels, including paid promotions with social media influencers. On one hand it is possible that such campaigns help destigmatise the concept of non-medical egg freezing and accelerate the social acceptance of fertility preservation. But on the other hand, there are growing concerns about the message provided and whether it is more persuasive than it is neutrally informational, which could compromise informed consent.

Beyond questions of impact and influence, van de Wiel (2020) argues that the advent of these clinics contributes in part to the growing commercialisation of the fertility sector. van de Wiel outlines a shift in the industry's focus from reproduction to that of proactive fertility preservation and expanding the pool of (potential) ART patients. Through campaigns that encourage younger women to take advantage of their fertility now, clinics appeal to individuals who do not want to risk childlessness in the future and encourage early intervention — which not only may be unnecessary, but also positions those who do undergo the procedure for further intervention in the future. Furthermore, many of the private companies offering egg freezing also give the option of managing the procedure costs through loans and subscription plans, thereby increasing patient numbers by facilitating access for those who may not otherwise have been able to afford the full cost out-of-pocket, while also increasing profit margins through loan interest rates.

While the development of schemes such as employer-sponsored egg freezing, *Freeze and Share* and commercial egg freezing companies have been proposed as a means to democratise access to egg freezing and empower women, they remain ethically ambiguous with unresolved concerns regarding what effect these developments may have on individuals and society more broadly. Some concerns include whether people are receiving adequate information to inform their decision making, what impact outsourcing procedure costs to employers will have on a person's reproductive autonomy and consent, and if these options enable broader access or further exacerbate socioeconomic disparities and encourage unnecessary intervention. Critically examining all these concerns is beyond the scope of this chapter. Rather these examples are described to demonstrate how alternative schemes have surfaced to fill the gap between high treatment costs and inadequate healthcare funding. While these schemes may indeed deliver on their promise to facilitate access to egg freezing (for certain people), the benefits of engaging in these schemes need to be considered in light of the potential harms.

11.3 Arguments for and Against Public Funding

In the previous sections we have outlined the different funding schemes that have been implemented to assist people to access egg freezing and we have discussed some of the common concerns that arise in response to the commercialisation of egg freezing. In this section we will consider the question of whether egg freezing should be publicly funded. Although relevant to this discussion, we do not consider the exact structure funding policies should take (e.g., full vs partial coverage or the timing of reimbursement) as they are likely to be influenced by existing local legal and economic factors (see Mertes and Pennings, 2012).

We will describe the most important arguments for and against funding, along with an examination of the crucial ethical issues. The value of reproductive autonomy (i.e., the basic right to decide freely if and when to reproduce) is often mentioned in the egg freezing debate but is *de facto* silent on the question of whether women are entitled to funding (Harwood, 2009). Theorists have, therefore, invoked other values, such as utility, social justice, equality and medical need to provide some more concrete guidance for determining how we should allocate funding resources. However, tensions between those values create ambiguity related to whether this procedure should be publicly funded.

11.3.1 Preserving the Chance of (Genetic) Parenthood

Procreation and parenting are generally accepted to be liberty but not claim rights; persons wishing to reproduce should be free to do so without interference, but this does not generate an obligation for any particular party (e.g., another person, organisation, the state, etc.) to assist them in fulfilling this right (Shanner, 1995). Despite this, in many jurisdictions assistance is provided, through the provision of public funding, to access ARTs. The availability of public funding for ART treatment is underpinned by the well-accepted view that having children is a significant life goal for many and contributes to increased well-being and life satisfaction. Hence, actions taken to preserve the chance of *future* parenthood, i.e., through freezing eggs to be used at a later date, could be seen as compatible with actions taken to facilitate parenthood in the present.

However, there are concerns about the broader social impacts that may arise from funding egg freezing. First, akin to the early debates regarding funding IVF, there are concerns that publicly funding egg freezing could reinforce pronatalist views (i.e., a social pressure to gestational motherhood) and geneticism (i.e., a social bias in favour of genetic motherhood) (Petropanagos, 2017). These social forces could shape the choice of egg freezing and result in coercively promoting and encouraging this option. This in turn could unduly undermine women's reproductive autonomy as well as make the choice of being childfree less acceptable.

Second, increasing public investment in ARTs may suggest that the state is not neutral between different means of satisfying the desire of parenthood and unduly privileges genetic opportunities over others (McTernan, 2015). There have been strong arguments that *genetic* motherhood should not be assumed to be a basic and core component of parenthood. Further, it has been argued that many of the reasons given in preference for genetic parenthood can be dismissed or can be satisfied through non-genetic forms of parenthood (Rulli, 2016).

To combat these concerns, efforts are needed to reduce social pressures in favour of genetic and gestational motherhood that may unduly compel women to utilise ARTs, including egg freezing. One way this could be addressed, at least partially, is to improve access to alternative pathways to parenthood such as adoption, fostering, or donor gametes (all of which are notoriously difficult and/or expensive to access) through interventions in policy. Ensuring these options are available, alongside that of ARTs (using genetic material) and promoting a position that life without children can be meaningful, may help ensure that reproductive autonomy is promoted and not undermined, and better serve well-being and life satisfaction, than expanding funding to egg freezing.

11.3.2 Efficacy, Cost-effectiveness, and the 'Value' of Egg Freezing

Questions of efficacy and cost-effectiveness are an important part of health care funding considerations. Generally, before a health intervention is subsidised, it is required to demonstrate cost effectiveness; this is to ensure public investment is worthwhile and the intervention produces the desired outcome, generating genuine personal and population benefits. In many nations, public funding is available for ARTs, so presumably the cost-effectiveness criterion has been satisfied, to at least some degree. However, as mentioned earlier, the shift in the timing of parenthood means many are now pursuing childbearing later in life. This has biological and (likely) financial repercussions. Age and fertility are inversely related, meaning the chance of conceiving either without assistance or through ART treatment at advanced ages is low. In addition, it is likely that those seeking ART treatment at older ages will require multiple cycles to collect a sufficient reserve of eggs. Taken together, pursuing ARTs (including egg freezing at advanced maternal ages) is not only less efficacious, but it is likely to require significant financial investment, thereby reducing overall cost effectiveness, in comparison to childbearing at younger ages.

Egg freezing may improve the likelihood of later childbearing. If egg freezing was accessed by individuals at younger ages (ideally between the ages of 30–35), not only would these eggs be of higher quality and thus more likely to lead to a viable pregnancy, but it is also likely that fewer cycles will be needed to collect a sufficient number of eggs. Therefore, providing financial support to assist people to access egg freezing when they are younger may be a more efficacious and cost-effective approach to facilitating childbearing later in life.

However, while in theory this seems valid, in practice this has yet to be demonstrated. Current reports indicate that rate of return following egg freezing ranges between 0–38% (Walker et al, 2023). Given this low rate of return, funding egg freezing (non-medical in particular) may not be a cost-effective investment since the majority do not require their banked eggs later in life. While there may be some validity to this objection, it rests on rate of return being the key factor when considering if egg freezing is a worthwhile public investment. But a question could be raised as to whether rate of return is the most appropriate or only relevant factor to measure whether egg freezing is a worthwhile investment. We know that most women who undergo egg freezing do so as a pre-emptive, precautionary measure if they are unable to conceive without assistance in the future. Meaning, their intention at the time of freezing is not to return to use their frozen eggs unless they are needed as a last resort. Furthermore, the benefit of egg freezing is not just limited to using eggs in future attempts at conception. Women who have frozen their eggs feel a sense of increased reproductive control and flexibility (Baldwin, 2018), clearly suggesting that egg freezing can provide substantial psychosocial benefits that are less easily quantified in monetary terms. The fact that those who freeze their eggs do so not with the intention of using them, and that the act of egg freezing can generate benefits beyond just future conception, challenges the validity of measuring cost-effectiveness and thus the value of egg freezing on rate of return alone.

Beyond questions of personal use, the fate of unused or 'surplus' eggs is an important factor to weigh into funding considerations and the 'value' of egg freezing. In many jurisdictions, when individuals have embryos or gametes surplus, they are offered the choice between discarding or donating (to research or reproduction). Subsequently, it is not unreasonable to imagine that if these surplus eggs are donated, either for research or reproductive pursuits of others, not only would the eggs not be wasted but there could also be tangible benefits for the community in terms of research advancement and helping others conceive (Pennings, 2023). Early indications suggest that very few decide to donate surplus eggs (Johnston et al, 2023). However as one of the authors has argued, there could be external barriers to preventing donation (Johnston et al, 2023). Only when barriers to donation are mitigated or ameliorated will we have a true understanding of the utility of unused frozen eggs.

11.3.3 Social (In)justice

Another argument in support of funding egg freezing is that it could work to democratise access (Cascante, 2023). Early reports of the demographics of women undergoing egg freezing (non-medical in particular) describe the majority as highly educated, working professionals on high incomes (Baldwin, 2015). Given these demographics, it is likely that procedural costs remain prohibitive for many who cannot afford to self-fund the procedure. Women who have frozen eggs themselves have argued that the restrictions on egg freezing coverage are unfair and discriminatory for other women (De Proost et al, 2022). While disparities in use are not uncommon and in some cases are unavoidable, what is important to consider is whether the factors that contribute to these disparities demonstrate inequity. Ability to pay is one factor that clearly contributes to disparities in use and is unacceptable if it is agreed that the decision to have children should not depend on income. For nations that already financially support ARTs, it is reasonable to presume that ability to pay is considered important when it comes to procreation. Therefore, if financial support was extended to include egg freezing, it could play a role in dismantling some of the barriers to fertility preservation, making it more accessible to a wider range of potential users and promoting equity of access.

On the other hand, one can assert that funding for egg freezing does not speak directly to structural injustices as there is no evidence that providing funding is enough to achieve social justice and equality in reproductive decision making (Pennings, 2021). A reproductive justice lens would likely focus on eliminating structural causes of unintended childlessness rather than inequality of access to egg freezing. Moreover, one could question that funding egg freezing would even further increase injustice rather than eliminate it. Access to fertility care is socially stratified, with low-income or women of colour being less likely to initiate such a procedure relative to more privileged women (De Proost & Coene, 2019). Such inequality in outcome has been referred to as a Matthew effect (a social phenomenon that describes how success breeds more success and failure breeds more failure – named for the parable of the Talents in St Matthew's gospel); here it is the observation that the benefits of government spending on funding ARTs disproportionally accrue to middle- and upper-class women. As such, investing in funding egg freezing runs the risk of increasing the gap among women and might reinforce existing inequalities rather than mitigating them.

11.3.4 Medicalisation

There may also be concerns that publicly funding (non-medical) egg freezing could encourage people to undergo the procedure unnecessarily, promoting unwarranted medical intervention for a problem that some argue is not medical, but social — namely reproductive aging and the postponement of women's first childbirth (Shkedi-Rafid & Hashiloni-Dolev, 2011). Instead of being seen as part of a natural life process, the onset of menopause and thus infertility is pathologised through the promotion of fertility preservation which transforms otherwise healthy women into patients obligated to seek medical help. As touched on earlier, the promotion of egg freezing by commercial clinics increases the risk of medicalisation through advertising egg freezing as a 'proactive' action in response to age. Further, egg freezing sets people up for later medical intervention if their frozen eggs are required for conception.

While concerns of the medicalisation of egg freezing is something that does warrant consideration, it needs to be done with an understanding of what the procedure of egg freezing entails. Egg freezing is invasive, onerous and is a physically as well as emotionally taxing procedure. It involves self-administrating daily hormone injections that can cause discomfort. In addition, there are some risks associated with hormonal stimulation, such as ovarian hyperstimulation syndrome, and while symptoms can vary from mild abdominal pain, bloating to nausea, in severe cases ovarian hyperstimulation syndrome can require hospitalisation and even result in death. Modern stimulation regimes have effectively eliminated the risk of severe ovarian hyperstimulation syndrome but no medical procedure is entirely risk free. Given these burdens and risks, it is not unrealistic to presume that people will weigh up the risks of egg freezing and how they fare in comparison to their circumstances and parenting desires, prior to undergoing the procedure. Concerns around people not being able to make an autonomous choice to undergo egg freezing is not a reason to restrict or reject support for access to egg freezing; doing so may be overly paternalistic. Rather these concerns create an imperative for the industry to ensure that people interested in egg freezing are provided with the information they need to make an informed decision.

There may also be benefits to the medicalisation of reproductive aging by means of fertility preservation. The understanding of egg freezing as medically necessary instead of a lifestyle choice may lead to positive outcomes such as improved normalisation of single parenting and the reduction in shame and stigmatisation associated with an inability to find a partner with whom to procreate.

11.3.5 Scarce Resources

Another important consideration to the question of funding egg freezing, is how to manage finite financial resources. The way resource distribution is managed is notoriously contested and it is a matter of debate as to which criteria are relevant in granting access to one person over another. While empirical data such as treatment efficacy or cost effectiveness may determine the most efficient way to distribute resources, it may not represent the fairest way. Affordability directly influences accessibility, therefore the criteria used to distribute funding has a direct impact on who can access what, and thus can have implications for social justice. Many funding policies already ration funding, and as described earlier, most currently use the distinction between 'medical' vs 'non-medical' egg freezing to distribute funding, with 'medical' cases awarded priority. For individuals who lack a medical indication, while they are still able to request egg freezing, their ability to access it is heavily dependent on whether they are able to afford the full costs.

In many instances, the medical/non-medical distinction is regarded as an almost self-evident justification to determine where health dollars are prioritised. Underlying the use of this distinction is the implicit assumption that medical needs are a greater or a more justified reason to access medical interventions in comparison to non-medical needs. This assumption is composed of two parts; first that a distinction between what constitutes as medical or non-medical can be determined; and second that this difference is morally relevant. However, as we have argued elsewhere, what qualifies as a legitimate 'medical' indication for egg freezing varies between jurisdictions, demonstrating there is no consensus on what constitutes a true 'medical' indication (De Proost and Johnston, 2021). Further, it is unclear whether age-related fertility decline should be categorised as a 'non-medical' threat to fertility or whether the attrition of fertility because of age justifies access to funding, like the loss of fertility from gonadotoxic treatments generally does. Resolving these questions is outside the scope of this chapter; however, given the challenges to the medical/non-medical distinction, there is a need for careful consideration as to whether this is the best criterion in which to use to distribute funding. If a morally relevant difference cannot be drawn between 'medical' and 'non-medical' egg freezing, then the justification for funding one over the other should be questioned.

As a final point, beyond how to distribute resources is the question of whether preserving a chance at genetic parenthood is enough of a compelling reason to dedicate limited healthcare dollars. One might claim that egg freezing should not be funded at all, given that health budgets are already strained and doing so could divert funds away from other reproductive interventions. Some have argued that the desire for genetic relatedness is a want not a need and that additional resources would be better allocated in ways that benefit a greater number of people (e.g., addressing other health priorities or non-health needs such as food and shelter) (Baylis, 2017). While these arguments are not unique to the question of funding egg freezing, they are important to consider as they prompt us to view resource distribution through a broader social justice lens.

11.4 Conclusion

After a decade of using egg freezing for an array of reasons, the question of funding is still on shaky moral ground. Given that the uptake of egg freezing is relatively recent, we do not know whether frozen eggs will deliver significant benefit for individual people and societies over a prolonged period. In this regard, it is remarkable that the current controversy on the issue of funding egg freezing reprises many of the assertions made initially against the public funding of IVF, such as its cost effectiveness and whether it is a form of unnecessary medicalisation. Furthermore, balancing costs and benefits is highly complex due to several unknown factors that introduces largely grey zones of what could be acceptable and unacceptable in funding of egg freezing. If some years from now it would turn out that very few people come back to use their eggs and that surplus eggs are not distributed for the benefit of research or others, it might be preferential to not prioritise funding for egg freezing. On the other hand, in jurisdictions that already offer generous funding for ARTs, extending funding to include egg freezing seems pragmatically consistent with the underlying rationale to support people in realising their goal to have genetically related children. Nonetheless, given the prohibitive costs associated with egg freezing, the availability of funding is likely to influence for who and under which circumstances access to egg freezing is supported. Therefore, if funding is provided, careful consideration is needed to determine which criteria should be used to distribute funding to ensure this is done in a coherent and fair manner.

References

Beaujouan É, Sobotka T. Is 40 the new 30? Increasing reproductive intentions and fertility rates beyond age 40. In: Nikolaou DS, Seifer DB, editors. Optimizing the management of fertility in women over 40. Cambridge University Press; 2020. p. 3–18.

Baldwin K. Conceptualising women's motivations for social egg freezing and experience of reproductive delay. Sociol Health Illn. 2018 Jun; 40(5):859–73.

Baldwin K, Culley L, Hudson N, Mitchell H, Lavery S. Oocyte cryopreservation for social reasons: Demographic profile and disposal intentions of UK users. Reprod Biomed Online. 2015 Aug;31(2): 239–45.

Baylis F. Human nuclear genome transfer (so-called mitochondrial replacement): Clearing the underbrush. Bioethics. 2017 Jan;31(1):7–19.

Calhaz-Jorge C, De Geyter CH, Kupka MS, Wyns C, Mocanu E, Motrenko T, Scaravelli G, Smeenk J, Vidakovic S, Goossens V. Survey on ART and IUI: legislation, regulation, funding and registries in European countries: The European IVF-monitoring Consortium (EIM) for the European Society of Human Reproduction and Embryology (ESHRE). Hum Reprod Open. 2020 Feb 6;2020(1):hoz044.

Cascante SD, Berkeley AS, Licciardi F, McCaffrey C, Grifo JA. Planned oocyte cryopreservation: The state of the ART. Reprod Biomed Online. 2023 Dec;47(6):103367.

Dash I, Pearce BCS, Armstrong S, Saunders C, Pacey A. Fertility preservation for women undergoing breast cancer treatment: A postcode lottery? Breast J. 2020 Oct;26(10):2117–8.

De Proost M, Coene G, Nekkebroeck J, Provoost V. 'I feel that injustice is being done to me': A qualitative study of women's viewpoints on the (lack of) reimbursement for social egg freezing. BMC Med Ethics. 2022 Mar 29;23(1):35.

De Proost M, Coene G. Emancipation on thin ice: Women's autonomy, reproductive justice, and social egg freezing. Tijdschrift voor Genderstudies. 2019 Nov;22(4):357–71.

De Proost M, Johnston M. The revision of the French bioethics law and the questions it raises for the future of funding for egg freezing. Reprod Biomed Online. 2022 Apr;44(4):591–3.

Dowling E. New survey finds employers adding fertility benefits to promote DEI [Internet]. Mercer; 2021. Available from: https://www.mercer.com/en-us/insights/us-health-news/new-survey-finds-employers-adding-fertility-benefits-to-promote-dei/

Harwood K. Egg freezing: A breakthrough for reproductive autonomy? Bioethics. 2009 Jan;23(1):39–46.

Human Fertilisation & Embryology Authority. Fertility treatment 2014 Trends and figures [Internet]. HFEA; 2016. Available from: http://www.hfea.gov.uk/docs/HFEA_Fertility_treatment_Trends_and_figures_2014.pdf.

Inhorn MC. Motherhood on ice: The mating gap and why women freeze their eggs. New York University Press; 2023.

Johnston M, Fuscaldo G, Sutton E, Hunt S, Zander-Fox D, Rombauts L, Mills C. Storage trends, usage and disposition outcomes following egg freezing. Reprod Biomed Online. 2023 Nov 16;48(4):103728.

Johnston M, Fuscaldo G, Gwini SM, Catt S, Richings NM. Financing future fertility: Women's views on funding egg freezing. Reprod Biomed Soc Online. 2021 Aug 13;14:32–41.

Johnston M, Fuscaldo G, Richings NM, Gwini SM, Catt S. Employer-sponsored egg freezing: Carrot or stick? AJOB Empir Bioeth. 2022 Jan–Mar;13(1):33–47.

McTernan E. Should fertility treatment be state funded?. Journal of Applied Philosophy. 2015;32(3):227–40.

Mertes H, Pennings G. Elective oocyte cryopreservation: Who should pay? Hum Reprod. 2012 Jan;27(1):9–13.

Miner SA, Miller WK, Grady C, Berkman BE. "It's just another added benefit": Women's experiences with employment-based egg freezing programs. AJOB Empir Bioeth. 2021 Jan-Mar;12(1):41–52.

Pennings G. When elective egg freezers become egg donors: Practical and ethical issues. Reprod Biomed Online. 2023 Jul;47(1):151–6.

Pennings G. Elective egg freezing and women's emancipation. Reprod Biomed Online. 2021 Jun;42(6):1053–5.

Petropanagos A. Pronatalism, geneticism, and ART. Int J Fem Approaches Bioeth. 2017;10(1):119–47.

Rulli T. Preferring a genetically-related child. J Moral Philos. 2016;13(6):669–98.

Shanner L. The right to procreate: When rights claims have gone wrong. McGill Law J. 1995 Aug;40(4):823–74.

Shkedi-Rafid S, Hashiloni-Dolev Y. Egg freezing for age-related fertility decline: Preventive medicine or a further medicalization of reproduction? Analyzing the new Israeli policy. Fertil Steril. 2011 Aug;96(2):291–4.

Shenfield F, de Mouzon J, Scaravelli G, Kupka M, Ferraretti AP, Prados FJ, Goossens V. Oocyte and ovarian tissue cryopreservation in European countries: Statutory background, practice, storage and use. Hum Reprod Open. 2017 Mar 29;2017(1):hox003.

van de Wiel L. The speculative turn in IVF: Egg freezing and the financialization of fertility. New Genetics and Society. 2020;39(3):306–26.

Walker Z, Lanes A, Ginsburg E. Oocyte cryopreservation review: Outcomes of medical oocyte cryopreservation and planned oocyte cryopreservation. Reprod Biol Endocrinol. 2022 Jan 7;20(1):10.

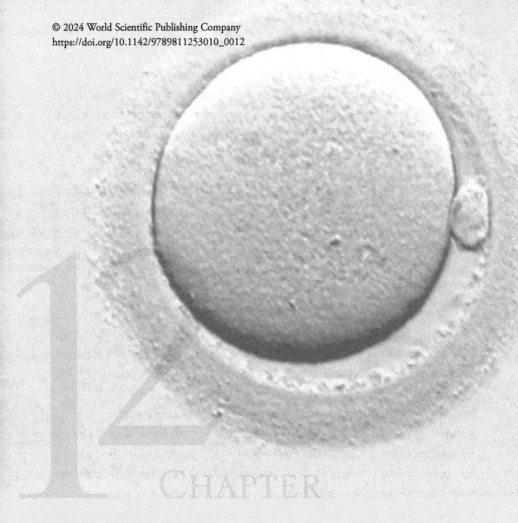

CHAPTER

Egg Donation:
The Future is Frozen

Nick Macklon, V Pataia and K Ahuja

Oocyte donation is now established as an effective fertility treatment for women of advanced reproductive age, for those with previous failed autologous treatment attempts, primary ovarian insufficiency, at risk of transmitting genetic conditions, and for male same-sex couples undergoing surrogacy. The UK has seen a remarkable increase in the number of oocyte donation cycles from around 2,000 to 4,400 per year between 2008 and 2019 (Human Fertilisation and Embryology Authority, 2019a). The effectiveness of egg donation is illustrated by a reported overall live birth rate (LBR) per embryo transfer of more than 25% for recipients of oocyte donation of any age in 2018, which compares favourably with a LBR per embryo transfer of 23% for all *in vitro* fertilisation (IVF) patients in the same period (Human Fertilisation and Embryology Authority, 2020). Other data sources indicate that the technique can achieve better outcomes. A recent UK registry study of treatment cycles using slow-frozen and vitrified donor oocytes between 2000–2016 reported a LBR per cycle of 30.7% (Mascarenhas et al, 2020).

There is good evidence that embryos, blastocysts and oocytes survive in greater numbers after vitrification than after slow freezing (Rienzi et al, 2017). Evidence in support of this remarkable observation has been strong enough to cause a decade-long increase in treatments with frozen embryos in autologous cycles and frozen eggs and embryos in autologous and heterologous cycles. This visible shift in approach is now reflected in three publications of recent registry data — from the USA (CDC, 2016), Japan (Isihara et al, 2019) and the UK (Human Fertilisation and Embryology Authority, 2019a) — in which the uptake of vitrification is evident in IVF and intracytoplasmic sperm injection, and in the continuing widespread use of preimplantation genetic testing for aneuploidy.

While vitrification is now well established as the gold standard method for oocyte cryopreservation due to its reliability and efficiency (Cornet-Bartolomé et al, 2020), it has taken some time for sufficient confidence in its reliability to grow to a point whereby eggs obtained from donors could be subject to this technique. However, the potential advantages for egg donation program providers, donors and recipients have long been clear.

12.1 The Impact of Vitrification

The national figures from the USA and Japan show quite clearly how the widespread introduction of vitrification has had such a revolutionary effect on assisted reproductive technologies, both in the cryopreservation of embryos and blastocysts and also of oocytes. But vitrification has had a 'disruptive' effect on the entire landscape of reproductive medicine (Ahuja and Macklon, 2020).

First, oocyte vitrification was given wider clinical direction in studies from Spain and Italy (where embryo freezing remained outlawed), with results showing clearly that delivery rates from frozen oocytes were reliable and consistent with those derived from fresh cycles (Rienzi et al, 2012). The authors' recommendation — that oocyte vitrification 'should be applied routinely for various indications' — has now been applied with vigour, and will very quickly become the default standard practice in egg donation. For egg donation patients, the advantages are clear — no need for overseas travel in search of donor eggs, no need to wait for a suitable donor or for synchronised cycles, a greater choice of donor, and a more efficient programme at lower cost. Moreover, oocyte vitrification has become a standard means of offering fertility preservation to women undergoing gonadotoxic medical treatments, for addressing uncertainty as to the likely duration of fertile years, and in other situations which argue for immediate recourse to IVF without immediate plans for pregnancy, such as the treatment of autoimmune conditions.

Despite a less than robust evidence base in its favour, there has nevertheless been a rapid shift towards the adoption of elective frozen embryo transfer cycles in routine IVF treatment (Acharya et al, 2018). The shift to frozen eggs in third-party egg donation has been even more striking. In the USA, the number of egg donation cycles from frozen donor eggs now far outstrips the numbers from fresh eggs

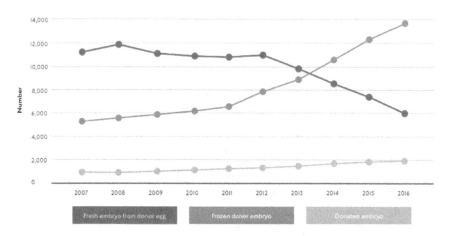

Figure 12.1 Number of assisted reproductive technology cycles using donor eggs 2007–2016. Reproduced with permission from Centers for Disease Control and Prevention, American Society for Reproductive Technology 2016 Assisted Reproductive Technology National Summary Report.

(Figure 12.1), with delivery rates not far different from those achieved in synchronised fresh treatments.

Similarly in Spain, where all clinics from 2016 were required by law to submit their data to a national registry run by the Spanish Fertility Society, 18% of all oocytes collected for egg donation treatments in 2016 were vitrified for egg banking, a total of more than 11,000 oocytes (www.registrosef.com/bulic/docs/sef2016). Significantly, egg donation (from fresh and frozen embryos) represented 53.3% of all of Spain's cross-border activity in 2016 (which totalled almost 13,000 cycles, about 10% of overall activity in which 138,553 cycles were recorded).

The rapid uptake of vitrification and egg banking has made cross-border transport of cryopreserved eggs feasible. Some Spanish clinics have already devised new cross-border arrangements in egg donation such that the gametes (and embryos) and not the patients do the travelling (La Marca et al, 2018). One strategy reported is based on shipping frozen sperm from the country of the recipient (Italy) to the country of the egg donor (Spain). Here, the thawed sperm is used to fertilise fresh oocytes collected from the donor and the resulting embryos are then frozen and shipped back to the referring IVF centre in Italy. A variation of this strategy, successfully introduced by another Spanish group, involved the shipment to Italy of vitrified oocytes rather than vitrified embryos (Parmegiani et al, 2019). Recent data from Italy, where the prohibition of gamete donation was removed in 2014 but where payment to gamete donors remains outlawed, show that gamete donation is still a minority activity of assisted reproductive technologies, and has not yet recovered from the draconian restrictions of Italy's 2004 Law 40. Indeed, in 2016 almost all cycles of cryopreserved oocyte donation were performed with oocytes from foreign banks (Figure 12.2) (http://old.iss.it/binary/rpmacont/executivesummaryofARTinITALYACTIVITY2016pdf).

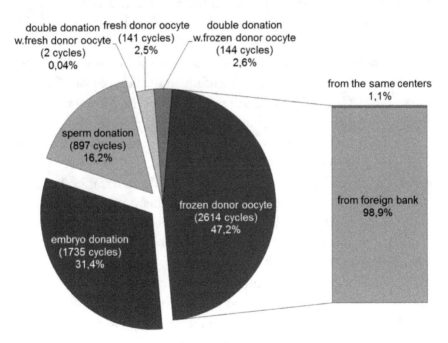

Figure 12.2   Distribution of all assisted reproductive technology cycles using donor gametes or cryopreserved embryos after donation and origin of the oocytes for the frozen donor oocyte cycles, 2016. Total cycles = 5533. Reproduced with permission from Registro Nazionale Procreazione Medicalmente Assistita — ISS, 2019.

Recently the clinical efficacy of an egg donation programme based on importing donated vitrified oocytes from cryo-banks located in a foreign country has been demonstrated (Scorio et al, 2021). In a retrospective study of 681 vitrified oocytes, survival rate after warming of 79% was reported, with fertilisation and blastulation rates of 90% and 48% respectively. Clinical pregnancy rate and LBR per embryo transfer were 31% and 28% respectively with a multiple pregnancy rate of <1%.

It was significant that the legal challenges to Italy's Law 40 came not from doctors but from patients, and significant too that court rulings were made in the interests of patients and not of the Italian lawmakers. Such patient pressure was similarly evident in the UK when the regulatory authority sought to resolve anomalies in gamete donation first by public consultation (in 2011) and later by a change in regulation (Ahuja, 2015). Until then, the UK had been critically unable to meet its own patient demands for donor sperm or donor eggs — with the result that donor sperm was almost exclusively imported and donor eggs only plentifully available in Spain, Cyprus, Ukraine and Czech Republic. After considering its consultation, the Human Fertilisation and Embryology Authority (HFEA) in April 2012 raised compensation to £35 'per visit' for sperm donors, and to £750 per cycle for oocyte donors; the revised fees, said the HFEA, should be viewed 'not in terms of crude sums but in terms of the value of donation'. The European Society of Human Reproduction and Embryology in 2011 had named 'fair access at home' as the most desirable circumstance of its cross-border good practice manual (Shenfield et al, 2011).

The effect of this publicly driven change was immediate and sustained, and coinciding with the growing confidence in egg vitrification, it caused a significant increase in the number of sperm and egg donors at many UK clinics. Accordingly, all gametes (male and female) for UK patients could now be supplied by donors recruited from within the UK. The need for overseas travel or imports for UK recipients is rapidly diminishing.

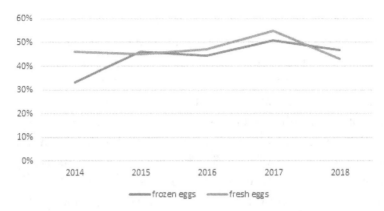

Figure 12.3   Clinical pregnancy live birth rates per embryo transfer at London Women's Clinic. Reproduced with permission from Ahuja and Macklon (2020).

This movement to greater patient autonomy in egg donation has now become even more pronounced with vitrification and frozen egg banking, which from 2014 gradually overtook overseas donation as the donor treatment of choice in our own clinic. Thus, of 1,283 donor cycles completed between 2005 and 2013, 88% were carried out at as cross-border treatments at overseas clinics. Since then, however, recognising the greater choice of frozen eggs available at home, 95% of patients have switched to 'home sourcing', compared with just 1% in 2013. The treatment is available without a waiting list for donor matching and the tedious need for synchronised cycles — and at lower cost. Moreover, overall pregnancy rates per transfer in our frozen egg programme are above 50%, matching those with fresh cycles (Figure 12.3).

12.2 Clinical Factors Determining Outcomes

A wide variation in ovarian response to gonadotrophin stimulation has been previously reported among healthy oocyte donors (Polyzos et al, 2012) and given the fine balance that must be achieved to obtain sufficient eggs to justify the intervention while minimising the burden of treatment to the donor, selection of the optimal type of stimulation is perhaps of even greater importance in the context of egg donation than in routine IVF (Rodriguez and Polyzos, 2021). The importance of identifying factors that can reliably predict response in this context is clear. In a recent systematic review of 57 studies focused on the safety and efficacy of ovarian stimulation in oocyte donors, antral follicle count and anti-Müllerian hormone (AMH) levels correlated with ovarian response to stimulation but were poor discriminators of donors likely to show either impaired or excessive response (Martinez et al, 2021).

There are conflicting reports on the impact of donor age (Barton et al, 2010; Humphries et al, 2019; Polyzos et al, 2012) and body-mass index (BMI) (Cardozo et al, 2016; Martínez et al, 2017) on oocyte yield. Moreover, the impact of donor reproductive history on oocyte yield remains unclear. In the UK, the HFEA guidelines (Human Fertilisation and Embryology Authority, 2019b) require all anonymous oocyte donors to be between 18–35 years of age, primarily because of the increase in oocyte aneuploidy rate associated with advancing maternal age. This policy is supported by a study showing a lower cumulative LBR in recipients of oocytes from donors aged ≥35 years old than from younger donors (Wu et al, 2012). However, recent findings also suggest that younger women may have less favourable treatment outcomes. For example, women aged <25 undergoing IVF treatment have been reported to have lower cumulative LBRs than women aged 25–29, followed by women 30–34 years (Wu et al, 2012). Another study has found a particularly high embryonic aneuploidy rate (>40%) in women ≤23, further supporting these findings (Franasiak et al, 2014).

Conflicting evidence also exists on the impact of other donor-related factors such as BMI (Cardozo et al, 2016; Martínez et al, 2017), oocyte yield (Baker et al, 2015; Hariton et al, 2017; Hipp et al, 2020) and prior reproductive history (Faber et al, 1997; Hariton et al, 2017) on recipient pregnancy and LBR. Moreover, the association between donor AMH levels and recipient outcomes remains largely unexplored, with just one study reporting no association between donor AMH and recipient pregnancy outcome (Riggs et al, 2011). Similarly, the effect of recipient age (Paulson et al, 1997; Soares et al, 2005; Yeh et al, 2014), BMI (Martínez et al, 2017; Provost et al, 2016) and previous reproductive history (Hariton et al, 2017) on pregnancy and LBR from oocyte donation treatment remains unclear.

One male factor thought to influence pregnancy and LBR is age (de La Rochebrochard et al, 2006). A paternal age of over 40 years at the time of conception is commonly considered to represent advanced paternal age (Humm and Sakkas, 2013) and was the upper age limit for sperm donors set by the HFEA until December 2019.

We recently addressed these issues in a retrospective study of 494 donor oocyte vitrification cycles and 705 subsequent recipient embryo transfers at a UK-regulated egg bank (Pataia et al, 2021). Donor age and AMH were found to predict total oocyte yield and total mature oocyte yield. Neither donor BMI nor reproductive history were predictors of oocyte yield. Up to an AMH level of 39.9 pmol/L, increasing AMH levels predicted higher total oocyte yield and mature oocyte yield. As might be anticipated, donors aged 30–35 had lower oocyte yield than donors 18–24 within the same AMH range of 15–29.9 pmol/L. In recipients, the rate of transferrable embryos per oocytes received, rate of transferrable embryos per oocytes fertilised, and number of embryo transfers needed to achieve the intended primary outcome were predictors of cumulative clinical pregnancy rate and LBR. Recipient BMI and previous miscarriages were predictors of cumulative LBR. Interestingly, donor age 18–22 was associated with a lower incidence of recipient clinical pregnancy and live birth after the first embryo transfer, as compared with donor age 23–29. However, no differences were found between recipients of donors aged 23–29 and 30–35. No other donor factors or paternal age were found to influence recipient outcomes. Since this first report of poorer outcomes associated with the use of vitrified oocytes from the youngest donors, other studies have described a similar phenomenon, which has been linked to a higher rate of aneuploidy in this age group compared to women in reproductive midlife.

A recent systematic review was unable to identify whether a particular type of gonadotrophin showed better outcomes when used for ovarian stimulation for egg donation due to the degree of heterogeneity between the five available randomized controlled trials (Martinez et al, 2021). No difference in ovarian response was evident comparing the use of gonadotropin-releasing hormone (GnRH) antagonists versus GnRH agonists to prevent premature luteinisation. Recently it has been proposed that progesterone treatment may represent a cheaper and simpler means of preventing premature luteinisation in this context than GnRH antagonist. The analysis of seven studies showed little or no difference between the two in mean number of retrieved oocytes or clinical pregnancy rates among recipients. With regard to triggering of final oocyte maturation, GnRH agonist is the gold standard and is recommended for use in all oocyte donors given the practical elimination of ovarian hyperstimulation syndrome risk. The systematic review showed no differences in number of mature eggs obtained or in pregnancy rates in recipients when the GnRH agonist trigger was compared to human chorionic gonadotropin. Importantly this review confirmed that the use of a levonorgestrel intrauterine device or a progestin contraceptive pill during ovarian stimulation did not impact the number of oocytes retrieved nor the clinical pregnancy rate in recipients. Finally, and particularly germane to the topic of this chapter, the use of fresh versus vitrified donated oocytes yielded similar pregnancy outcomes (Martinez et al, 2021).

12.3 Safety of Oocyte Vitrification

Given the stresses that vitrification places on oocytes, there has been some concern that despite the excellent pregnancy outcomes evident when using this approach, it may have longer-term consequences for the health of offspring. Reasons for concern arise because oocyte vitrification combines the use of high, possibly toxic, concentrations of cryoprotectants with ultra-rapid cooling rates, which may cause cryodamage to the oocytes (Cobo et al, 2014). The few studies that have investigated the safety of oocyte vitrification indicate that obstetric outcomes are reassuring. Moreover, the incidence of complications such as antepartum haemorrhage, pre-eclampsia and preterm delivery appear to be comparable between vitrified and fresh oocyte-derived pregnancies (Cobo et al, 2014), while neonatal outcomes too are reported to be similar. To date, babies born after oocyte vitrification have shown no evidence of differing from other children in terms of mean birthweight APGAR scores (Seshadri et al, 2018) and risk of birth defects after conception from donor eggs (Cobo et al, 2014). These data have led to the Practice Committee of the American Society for Reproductive Medicine advising that using vitrified oocytes is not associated with increased perinatal risks (Practice Committee of the American Society for Reproductive Medicine, 2013). A recent study has extended the period of follow-up to investigate how two-year-old children compare with peers born after use of fresh oocytes in a donation programme (van Reckem, 2021). Biometric parameters including weight, BMI, and head circumference together with rates of hospital admission and surgical interventions were compared between 72 two-year-old children born after oocyte vitrification and 41 born after use of fresh donor oocytes. None of these endpoints differed significantly between the two groups of children. While prospective data from larger cohorts are required to confirm these observations, there is at present no evidence to indicate a need for concern about the increasingly prevalent use of vitrified oocytes in this context.

12.4 Egg Donation: Is the Future Frozen?

Oocyte vitrification is profoundly affecting not only the techniques and logistics of egg donation but greatly increasing access, choice and convenience. To date the evidence base relating to efficacy and safety supports the increasing use of vitrified oocytes being observed (Ahuja and Macklon, 2020). However, long-term outcome data in children and adults born after this treatment are still awaited and follow-up and register studies are required to confirm its potential role as the future default means of providing oocytes to donor egg recipients.

References

Acharya KS, Acharya CR, Bishop K, Harris B, Raburn D, Muasher SJ. Freezing of all embryos in in vitro fertilization is beneficial in high responders, but not intermediate and low responders: An analysis of 82,935 cycles from the Society for Assisted Reproductive Technology registry. Fertil Steril. 2018;108:e390.

Ahuja KK, Macklon N. Vitrification and the demise of fresh treatment cycles in ART. Reprod Biomed Online. 2020;41:217–24.

Ahuja KK. Patient pressure: Is the tide of cross-border reproductive care beginning to turn? Reprod Biomed Online. 2015;30:447–50.

Baker VL, Brown MB, Luke B, Conrad KP. Association of number of retrieved oocytes with live birth rate and birth weight: An analysis of 231,815 cycles of in vitro fertilization. Fertil Steril. 2015;103:931–38.

Barton SE, Missmer SA, Ashby RK, Ginsburg ES. Multivariate analysis of the association between oocyte donor characteristics, including basal follicle stimulating hormone (FSH) and age, and IVF cycle outcomes. Fertil Steril. 2010;94:1292–5.

Cardozo ER, Karmon AE, Gold J, Petrozza JC, Styer AK. Reproductive outcomes in oocyte donation cycles are associated with donor BMI. Hum Reprod. 2016;31:385–92.

Center for Disease Control and Prevention, American Society for Reproductive Medicine, Society for Assisted Reproductive Technology. 2016 Assisted Reproductive Technology National Summary Report. https://www.cdc.gov/art/pdf/2016-report/art-2016-national-summary-report.pdf

Cobo A, Serra V, Garrido N, Olmo I, Pellicer A, Remohí J. Obstetric and perinatal outcome of babies born from vitrified oocytes. Fertil Steril. 2014;102:1006–15.

Cornet-Bartolomé D, Rodriguez A, García D, Barragán M, Vassena R. Efficiency and efficacy of vitrification in 35 654 sibling oocytes from donation cycles Hum Reprod. 2020 Oct 1;35(10):2262–71.

de La Rochebrochard E, de Mouzon J, Thépot F, Thonneau P. Fathers over 40 and increased failure to conceive: The lessons of in vitro fertilization in France. Fertil Steril. 2006;85:1420–4.

Faber BM, Muasher SJ, Mercan R, Toner JP, Harnacher P. The impact of an egg donor's age and her prior fertility on recipient pregnancy outcome. Fertil Steril. 1997;68:370–2.

Franasiak JM, Forman EJ, Hong KH, Werner MD, Upham KM, Treff NR, Scott RT. The nature of aneuploidy with increasing age of the female partner: A review of 15,169 consecutive trophectoderm biopsies evaluated with comprehensive chromosomal screening. Fertil Steril. 2014;101:656–63.

Hariton E, Kim K, Mumford SL, Palmor M, Bortoletto P, Cardozo ER, Karmon AE, Sabatini ME, Styer AK. Total number of oocytes and zygotes are predictive of live birth pregnancy in fresh donor oocyte in vitro fertilization cycles. Fertil Steril. 2017;108:262–8.

Hipp HS, Gaskins AJ, Nagy ZP, Capelouto SM, Shapiro DB, Spencer JB. Effect of oocyte donor stimulation on recipient outcomes: data from a US national donor oocyte bank. Hum Reprod. 2020;35:847–58.

Human Fertilisation and Embryology Authority, 2019a. Trends in egg and sperm donation. https://www.hfea.gov.uk/2019

Human Fertilisation and Embryology Authority, 2019b. Code of Practice 9th Edition. https://www.hfea.gov.uk/knowledge-base/read-the-code-of-practice

Human Fertilisation and Embryology Authority, 2020. Fertility treatment 2018: Trends and figures UK statistics for IVF and DI treatment, storage, and donation. https://ww.hfea.gov.uk/2018

Humm KC, Sakkas D. Role of increased male age in IVF and egg donation: Is sperm DNA fragmentation responsible? Fertil Steril. 2013 Jan; 99(1):30–6.

Humphries LA, Dodge LE, Kennedy EB, Humm KC, Hacker MR, Sakkas D. Is younger better? Donor age less than 25 does not predict more favorable outcomes after in vitro fertilization. J Assist Reprod Genet. 2019;36:1631–7.

Ishihara O, Jwa SC, Kuwahara A, Tomonori I, Koji K, Rintaro S, Kouji B, Minoru I, Hidekazu S. Assisted reproductive technology in Japan: A summary report for 2016 by the Ethics Committee of the Japan Society of Obstetrics and Gynecology. Reprod Med Biol. 2019;18:7–16.

La Marca A, Dal Canto M, Buccheri M, Valerio M, Mignini Renzini M, Rodriguez A, Vassena R. A novel transnational fresh oocyte donation (TOD) program based on transport of frozen sperm and embryos. Hum Reprod. 2018;34:285–90.

Martínez F, Kava-Braverman A, Clúa E, Rodríguez I, Gaggiotti Marre S, Coroleu B, Barri PN. Reproductive outcomes in recipients are not associated with oocyte donor body mass index up to 28 kg/m2: A cohort study of 2722 cycles. Reprod Biomed Online. 2017;35:739–46.

Martínez F, Racca A, Rodríguez I, Polyzos NP. Ovarian stimulation for oocyte donation: A systematic review and meta-analysis. Hum Reprod Update. 2021;27:673–96.

Mascarenhas M, Mehlawat H, Kirubakaran R, Bhandari H, Choudhary M. Live birth and perinatal outcomes using cryopreserved oocytes: An analysis of the Human Fertilisation and Embryology Authority database from 2000 to 2016 using three clinical models. Hum Reprod. 2021;36:1416–26.

Parmegiani L, Quintero L, Filicori M. Transnational oocyte donation program: Fresh versus vitrified oocytes. Hum Reprod 2019;34:2551.

Pataia V, Nair S, Wolska M, Linara-Demakakou E, Shah T, Lamanna G, Macklon N, Ahuja KK. Factors predicting clinical outcomes from 494 vitrified oocyte donation cycles at a UK-regulated egg bank. Reprod Biomed Online. 2021 Sep;43(3):453–65.

Paulson RJ, Hatch IE, Lobo RA, Sauer MV. Cumulative conception and live birth rates after oocyte donation: Implications regarding endometrial receptivity. Hum Reprod. 1997;12:835–9.

Polyzos NP, Stoop D, Blockeel C, Adriaensen P, Platteau P, Anckaert E, Smitz J, Devroey P. Anti-Müllerian hormone for the assessment of ovarian response in GnRH-antagonist-treated oocyte donors. Reprod Biomed Online. 2012;24:532–9.

Practice Committee of American Society for Reproductive Medicine and Society for Assisted Reproductive Technology. Mature oocyte cryopreservation: A guideline. Fertil Steril. 2013;99:37–43.

Provost MP, Acharya KS, Acharya CR, Yeh JS, Steward RG, Eaton JL, Goldfarb JM, Muasher SJ. Pregnancy outcomes decline with increasing recipient body mass index: An analysis of 22,317 fresh donor/ recipient cycles from the 2008–2010 Society for Assisted Reproductive Technology Clinic Outcome Reporting System registry. Fertil Steril. 2016;105:364–8.

Rienzi L, Cobo A, Paffoni A, Scarduelli C, Capalbo A, Vajta G, Remohí J, Ragni G, Ubaldi FM. Consistent and predictable delivery rates after oocyte vitrification: An observational longitudinal cohort multicentric study. Hum Reprod. 2012;27:1606–12.

Rienzi L, Gracia C, Maggiulli R, LaBarbera AR, Kaser DJ, Ubaldi FM, Vanderpoel S, Racowsky C. Oocyte, embryo and blastocyst cryopreservation in ART: Systematic review and meta-analysis comparing slow-freezing versus vitrification to produce evidence for the development of global guidance. Hum Reprod Update. 2017;23:139–55.

Riggs R, Kimble T, Oehninger S, Bocca S, Zhao Y, Leader B, Stadtmauer L. Anti-Müllerian hormone serum levels predict response to controlled ovarian hyperstimulation but not embryo quality or pregnancy outcome in oocyte donation. Fertil Steril. 2011;95:410–2.

Scorio R, Antonini E, Engl B. Live birth and clinical outcome of vitrification-warming donor oocyte programme: An experience of a single IVF unit. Zygote. 2021;29:410–16.

Seshadri S, Saab W, Exeter H, Drew E, Petrie A, Davies M, Serhal P. Clinical outcomes of a vitrified donor oocyte programme: A single UK centre experience. Eur J Obstet Gynecol Reprod Biol. 2018;225:136–40.

Shenfield F, de Mouzon J, Pennings G, Ferraretti AP, Goossens V. ESHRE's good practice guide for cross-border reproductive care. Hum Reprod. 2011;26:1625–7.

Soares SR, Troncoso C, Bosch E, Serra V, Simón C, Remohí J, Pellicer A. Age and uterine receptiveness: Predicting the outcome of oocyte donation cycles. J Clin Endocrinol Metab. 2005;90:4399–404.

Van Reckem M, Blockeel C, Bonduelle M, Buysse A, Roelants M, Verheyen G, Tournaye H, Hes F, Belva F. Health of 2-year-old children born after vitrified oocyte donation in comparison with peers born after fresh oocyte donation. Hum Reprod Open. 2021;2021(1):hoab002.

Wu LH, Humm KC, Dodge LE, Sakkas D, Hacker MR, Penzias AS. IVF outcomes are paradoxically poorer under age 25. Fertil Steril. 2012;98:S264.

Yeh JS, Steward RG, Dude AM, Shah AA, Goldfarb JM, Muasher SJ. Pregnancy outcomes decline in recipients over age 44: An analysis of 27,959 fresh donor oocyte in vitro fertilization cycles from the Society for Assisted Reproductive Technology. Fertil Steril. 2014;101(5):1331–6.

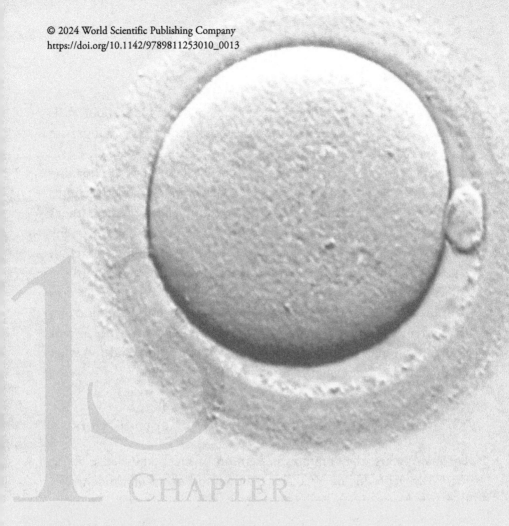

CHAPTER

Male Attitudes
to Oocyte Cryopreservation

Allan Pacey

13.1 Introduction

It is insightful of the Editor to commission a chapter about male attitudes to oocyte cryopreservation in a book about egg freezing. I am not sure that the many books about sperm freezing to date have ever given equal attention to the views of women. However, we are reaching a time where there is better gender equality in reproductive rights and so it does seem fitting. The chapter is influenced by the author's 30 years of service in Andrology, but also with reference to many authors of papers and reviews (for which I am most grateful). Therefore, by way of introduction, if we are to fully understand the subject of male attitudes to oocyte cryopreservation, then we need to consider four areas: (i) men's knowledge of their own reproduction; (ii) current fertility preservation methods for men; (iii) the current literature on male attitudes to oocyte cryopreservation; and (iv) what we do not know and what research needs to be done.

13.2 Men's Knowledge of their Own Reproduction

For many years, the common perception of men's knowledge about their own reproduction (let alone the reproduction of women) was that it was very poor, and they were largely uninterested. This was probably reinforced by many factors which include (but are not limited to) the fact that historically: (i) fertility issues have been mostly managed by gynaecologists (who by their very nature are more interested in the reproductive biology of women); (ii) fertility clinics were (and often still are) located in maternity hospitals (which by their very name are not welcoming places for men as patients); (iii) sex education in schools and higher education has been more frequently focussed around the prevention of unwanted pregnancy and avoidance of sexually transmitted infections rather than in preparing men and women for future fertility; and (iv) popular culture as seen on TV and in mainstream media have more frequently focussed on the infertility struggles of women rather than men (and where male fertility and sperm are often seen as a source of fun). Whilst these are on the one hand sweeping generalisations, on the other they represent a historical disparity on how fertility issues of men and women within our society have been framed and consequently how men may view the topic of oocyte cryopreservation.

To date, our academic knowledge about how well men understand their own reproduction has been limited by a general lack of empirical research on the subject. However, thankfully, in recent years this has been slowly changing. The most up-to-date evidence base which summarises men's knowledge about their fertility was published by Hammarberg et al (2017). This meta-analysis looked at 43 (mostly observational) unique studies conducted between 2005 and 2016 and concluded that although the studies conducted to date varied considerably in their design and approach, it was fair to conclude that men are indeed less knowledgeable about fertility issues compared to women. Fertility knowledge was generally better in men who were actively trying to conceive with their partner or in those men who had undertaken some fertility education. But it was poorer in young men and men from a low socioeconomic background. However, although men felt "fairly knowledgeable", when it was tested their fertility knowledge was quite low and they frequently over-estimated the chance of successful conception, either naturally or with assisted reproduction. Critically for this chapter, when they were specifically asked about the impact of age on women's fertility (given that this is a major influence on women's desire to freeze eggs) men were generally aware that it had an impact but compared to women they believed that it occurred at a much later age than it actually did.

In addition to men's fertility knowledge, Hammarberg et al (2017) also examined their attitudes to parenthood. Perhaps in contrast to the popular belief that men are uninterested in parenthood, many studies show that most men do indeed value it and both want and expect to become fathers. Perhaps surprisingly, studies seem to show that men would be upset if they were found to be infertile, disappointed if they did not become fathers, and feel that having children is important for life fulfilment and commitment. This has been confirmed with more recent studies which have shown that men in Sweden and Denmark wanted to have children in the future but felt there was a need to follow the "right order". By this they meant to first complete their education, get a good job and a good financial position, establish a stable and meaningful relationship before having children. Even then, they were heavily influenced by their social circle and were not always ready to give up their freedom, even when they felt mature enough to have children (Hviid et al, 2020). However, the desire of men to want children is not universal. In a study of Ukrainian (Russian-speaking) medical students, Mogilevkina et al (2016) reported that one in four males (25%) did not want to have children. Similarly, Kato (2018) examined the fertility intentions of 8,944 single, childless Japanese men and found that those who had a preference for sharing household and domestic duties in a more equal manner with their partner had very low fertility intentions (i.e., modern men were less interested in becoming fathers).

It is important to note that in understanding men's knowledge of fertility and their attitudes to future parenthood that most of our knowledge comes from studies which have taken place in high-income countries. Very few studies have examined the question in low- and middle-income countries, particularly in sub-Saharan Africa, where cultural norms can be quite different compared to those in the global north. However, a few studies do exist. For example, back in the 1980s Adamchak et al (1987) studied a sample of 202 male Nigerians enrolled in colleges and graduate schools in the USA (Kansas). Interestingly, 43% believed a man should divorce his wife if she was infertile, unable to produce a male child, or unable to bear the number of children he demanded. Furthermore, 35% suggested a man should marry a second wife, or continue to have children, if the couple has five daughters and no sons. The majority (62%) viewed children as wealth or better than wealth. Similarly, an interview study by Dierickx et al (2021) involving 13 men from different ethnic groups, locations, religions, backgrounds, and ages in The Gambia (West Africa) found men had a very poor knowledge of their fertility, often attributing any problems to God and spiritual powers or "blood incompatibility" with their partner. Infertility of all causes was frequently attributed to the female partner, thus exacerbating the historic normative gendered-based frameworks of reproduction.

Therefore, in the context of this chapter, it is important to recognise these views and country-level differences in the context of men's attitudes towards parenthood, and therefore their likely attitudes to oocyte cryopreservation.

13.3 Current Fertility Preservation Methods for Men

In comparison to women, fertility preservation for men through the freezing of ejaculated spermatozoa (the most comparable process to oocyte cryopreservation) has been available for over 70 years. The science and technology of sperm freezing was first developed in the 1950s and 60s with Sherman and Bunge (1953) and Perloff (1964) developing the techniques which formed the basis of modern sperm banks (and indeed paving the way for oocyte cryopreservation).

However, it was not really until the late 1970s that sperm banking became more widely available around the world although they were primarily located in tertiary centres such as large teaching hospitals and typically only offered their services to selected cancer patients as a way of preserving their fertility prior to radiotherapy or chemotherapy. This is crucial to understanding male attitudes to oocyte cryopreservation because even though banking sperm has been technically mainstream for 40 years, it has largely been out of plain sight of most males in the population unless they had a direct experience of cancer in themselves or a close friend or family member.

Even then, many studies have shown that sperm banking prior to cancer treatment is not always offered appropriately, either because of miscommunication between doctor and patient, assumptions made by healthcare professionals about the man's wishes, or because the man himself feels it is not for him and they would rather get on with their lifesaving treatment (Pacey and Eiser, 2011). The invisible nature of sperm banking is further compounded by the fact that of the many men who actually get the opportunity and agree to bank sperm, only a relative minority (often <10%) then ever need to use the frozen samples to achieve pregnancy with their partner (primarily because for a surprising number their fertility returns or they choose not to have children after their cancer experience). Thus, there is a general lack of popular narratives around the process and value of sperm banking for men and the benefits that it brings. Surely, this feeds into men's views about oocyte cryopreservation.

An alternative use for sperm banking is in the recruitment and supply of screened donor sperm for use in donor insemination or *in vitro* fertilisation (IVF) where donor gametes are also needed. Donor sperm banks flourished since the early 1980s, primarily driven by the HIV epidemic and the realisation that it could be transmitted via semen in a medical (as well as social) setting (Pacey, 2010). In the early 1990s there were many thousands of cycles of donor insemination in the United Kingdom and although this figure has subsequently fallen with the advent of intracytoplasmic sperm injection (ICSI), the use of donor sperm is still of major importance for the family formation of single women and same-sex couples (Hamilton et al, 2008). However, again, it is plausible that for the majority of men the existence of donor sperm banks probably has little impact on their understanding of oocyte cryopreservation because the use of donor sperm (at least in a heterosexual couple) is probably still a source of secrecy.

It is only in recent years that sperm cryopreservation for men's own social reasons has been debated. This has gained theoretical significance given the observations that older men are generally less fertile and the offspring of older fathers are statistically less healthy than children born to younger men (Pacey and Martins da Silva, 2020). It is for this reason that the upper age limits for sperm donors is capped at 40 years old (Pacey, 2010), although this fact is not relevant to the current chapter. But Smith (2015) first raised a debate about the potential value of social sperm freezing, by arguing that there should be appropriate health education to promote earlier fatherhood, as well as incentives for young sperm donors and the availability of state-supported universal sperm banking. He argued that sperm could be taken (on a voluntary basis) from all young men, with artificial insemination becoming the norm for procreation (later in life). However, although this was an eloquently argued opinion, it ignored the fact that given the variable quality of frozen-thawed sperm from men in the general population, intra-uterine insemination would not be successful for the majority, and it would therefore inevitably require widespread use of IVF (and/or ICSI) with the albeit small but associated risks of doing so being shouldered by the female partner (Pacey and Martins da Silva, 2020). Moreover, as Pennings et al (2021) pointed out, sperm freezing may itself cause damage to the genetic integrity of sperm, thus leading to the remedy of reproductive aging actually undoing the possible benefits in terms of fertility and health of any offspring born. To date there is not widespread uptake of social sperm freezing to guard against male age-related fertility decline. Typically, only men with very high-risk occupations (e.g., soldiers or policemen) ever take up the offer (and in the authors' experience this is a rare event). Therefore, apart from this limited group, most men probably have very little insight about their own fertility preservation options, let along those of women.

13.4 Male Attitudes to Oocyte Cryopreservation

Several studies have directly or indirectly examined men's knowledge of attitudes to oocyte cryopreservation, although these have largely been restricted to: (i) university students; (ii) medical professionals; or (iii) the general public.

Studies of university students include one conducted in Hannover (Germany) where Meissner et al (2016) obtained information from 1,144 German university students via an anonymous questionnaire. Somewhat surprisingly this found that 57% of male students and 54% of female students knew about the concept of oocyte freezing. However, when asked if they would like to have more information, only a relative minority (4% females and 0.8% males) said they would. A similar study by Hashiloni-Dolev et al (2020) examined the knowledge, concerns and intentions of Israeli and Danish students of both genders to fertility preservation. They found that 51% of Israeli and 62% of Danish men had heard of egg freezing and 11% and 13% had known someone who had undergone it. Both of these studies show that in these student populations at least, men had a surprisingly high awareness of oocyte cryopreservation, although with no obvious desire to know more.

With regard to medical professionals, the picture is more mixed. For example, Nasab et al (2019) examined the fertility knowledge and attitudes to oocyte cryopreservation of 350 medical professionals at the University of Texas. However, only a minority of respondents (27%) were male, making it almost impossible to understand their views. In a similar study of obstetrics and gynaecology residents in the USA (Yu et al, 2016) only 9.7% of respondents were males, meaning the study lacked sufficient power to understand their views compared to their female colleagues. Why male medical professionals were so reluctant to participate in these two studies is unclear, but it means we are missing an important perspective. Unfortunately, to the authors' knowledge, there are no studies of men's views about oocyte cryopreservation in other occupations.

Similarly, there have been relatively few studies that examined the perspective of male members of the general population to oocyte cryopreservation. However, a study by Lewis et al (2016), which examined a nationally representative sample of 1,064 people based on age, sex and race, found general support (72%) for oocyte cryopreservation because of "delayed childbearing for career enhancement", which was second only to support for "cancer patients" (89%), and behind "insufficient funds for child rearing" (58%). Interestingly, men were less supportive of women undergoing oocyte cryopreservation because they did not have a partner and for future use of cryopreserved oocytes without being married. This latter point is interesting, given that studies consistently show that one of the main drivers for women to undergo oocyte cryopreservation in the first place is because men often seem reluctant to commit to stable relationships and fatherhood.

Perhaps the most detailed investigation about men's participation (and therefore views) in women undergoing oocyte cryopreservation comes from the study by Marcia Inhorn (who is the author of another chapter in this book). She interviewed 114 women in the USA and 36 in Israel to establish whether men played supportive roles either before, during or after elective oocyte preservation (Inhorn et al, 2020). She described how nearly two-thirds of women relied on some kind of male support during elective oocyte cryopreservation. This included support from a range of different men including fathers (or father figures), male partners (past or present), male friends, brothers and in some instances male judges. The latter is a particularly interesting and surprising category, and the paper describes how increasingly in the USA some judges are ordering ex-husbands to pay for oocyte cryopreservation as part of divorce settlements. In total the paper identified four major categories of support given by men which included (i) instrumental (seeking information, attending appointments, etc.); (ii) financial; (iii) physical (assisting with injections or providing post-egg retrieval food and care, etc.); and (iv) psychological. Critically, this one paper does show that many different men can be very involved in oocyte cryopreservation, and at a number of different levels, although to the outside world their role may be somewhat hidden.

13.5 What We Do Not Know and What Research Needs to be Done

So far, this chapter has outlined how men have relatively limited understanding of fertility and reproductive biology compared to women. It also argues that although fertility preservation methods for males (i.e., sperm banking) have been around for many years, it is probably invisible to most men and therefore unlikely to shape their views about oocyte cryopreservation for women. In spite of this, the limited data that exist suggest that male university students, and to some extent men in the general population, are broadly supportive of oocyte cryopreservation. Moreover, in some instances men would seem to provide pivotal practical and supportive roles to women who choose to undergo oocyte cryopreservation for social reasons. However, it is fair to say that our understanding of men's attitudes to oocyte cryopreservation is fairly limited and many of these statements are generalisations from the current available literature (which is not vast). Moreover, since most studies suggest that the main driver for women electing to preserve their fertility is the lack of a suitable male partner (e.g., Inhorn et al, 2018), some of the observations feel slightly ironic. Therefore, the concluding sections of the chapter will outline two areas which in the authors' opinion require urgent attention: (i) increase male engagement with fertility issues generally; and (ii) increase male engagement with fertility research.

The suggestion that we need to increase male engagement with fertility issues generally comes from a couple of different perspectives. First, at the start of this chapter, it was outlined how historically men have often been either deliberately or inadvertently excluded from social narratives about reproductive health. In addition, it has been highlighted how healthcare structures in reproductive medicine are often not always male-friendly. For example, in a paper entitled "You did not turn up... I did not realise I was invited...: understanding male attitudes towards engagement in fertility and reproductive health discussions", Grace et al (2019) reported the results from 35 semi-structured telephone and face-to-face interviews with lay men and women as well as health professionals in the UK. She described how both men and women saw fertility as a woman's issue, but from very different viewpoints. Whilst men generally wanted to be involved in childbearing discussions, and improve their fertility knowledge, they felt they did not have a voice on the topic because discussions have traditionally focussed on women. She concluded that "the notion that men are not expected to be interested and engaged thus becomes a self-fulfilling prophecy". The paper concludes that concerted effort by charity organisations, educators, healthcare service providers, and policymakers are needed to proactively encourage male involvement in reproductive decision making. This includes the design of "male-inclusive reproductive health services". One of the important components of changing the narrative surrounding men's reproductive health is communication. Critically, in her 2014 book "Conceiving Masculinity" Liberty Barnes highlighted how there was an entire culture and medical system which makes it possible for men to be infertile and not realise it (Barnes, 2014). In addressing this, perhaps technology holds the key. In a study of 1,346 young people aged 13–18 in 10 UK schools from diverse socioeconomic areas, Goodyear and Quennerstedt (2019) found that one of the main reasons young men engaged with social media was to access health-related information. Moreover, irony and humour were central learning mechanisms and "acceptable banter" allowed them to engage with health discourses without fear of peer ridicule. These observations suggest that providing men with a safe environment to become involved in the dialogue may help shape their participation in reproduction and, perhaps over time, their attitudes to oocyte cryopreservation.

In terms of increasing men's engagement with fertility research, Grace et al (2019) also highlighted how in previous research studies relatively little attention had been given to men, but how also there was poor engagement by men as well as a dearth of information from, and on, the male perspective. She concluded that in trying to proactively encourage male involvement in reproductive decision making, it was also necessary to develop male-friendly research study design approaches. It has been known for some time that men have been marginalised in the social science literature on infertility (Culley et al, 2013) and the suggestion has been made that there is a need to reframe the research agenda on men and assisted reproduction. The same has been noted in studies concerning semen quality where significant recruitment bias and low participation rates can exist (Stewart et al, 2009). This means that even when men participate in studies, their opinions may not be representative. In a recent qualitative study of factors influencing male participation in fertility research, Harlow et al (2020) concluded that there was a need for more education and health communication on male fertility to normalise male participation in fertility and reproductive health research. They concluded that men are motivated to participate in infertility research to support their partners, to help others, and to learn more about their own reproductive health. Clearly, there needs to be renewed focus on undertaking research studies with men to understand their perspectives on fertility preservation and oocyte cryopreservation in particular.

13.6 Summary and Conclusions

In summary, our knowledge of men's attitudes to oocyte cryopreservation is still limited but we know enough to conclude that men are generally supportive of it and in some instances are actively involved. However, there is much more to learn about men's attitudes to fertility and at the heart of this is why they seem to delay their own commitment to parenthood, which is a major driver for women to need to undertake oocyte cryopreservation in the first place. It is curious that at the time of writing, there are only four countries in the world with a specific policy for men's health (Australia, Brazil, Iran, and Ireland) (Early and Devine, 2020). Whilst these policies do not directly tackle issues of male reproductive health and fertility, they set the scene for a broader framework about men's health and how seriously it is taken. Perhaps if other countries took male reproductive health more seriously, and had their own policies on men's health, many of the issues raised in this chapter about men's views on oocyte cryopreservation would be better understood and solutions be more firmly in our grasp.

References

Adamchak DJ, Adebayo A. Male fertility attitudes: A neglected dimension in Nigerian fertility research. Soc Biol. 1987;34(1–2):57–67.

Barnes LW. Conceiving masculinity: Male infertility, medicine, and identity. Temple University Press; 2014.

Culley L, Hudson N, Lohan M. Where are all the men? The marginalization of men in social scientific research on infertility. Reprod Biomed Online. 2013;27(3):225–35.

Dierickx S, Oruko KO, Clarke E, Ceesay S, Pacey A, Balen J. Men and infertility in The Gambia: Limited biomedical knowledge and awareness discourage male involvement and exacerbate gender-based impacts of infertility. PLoS One. 2021;16(11):e0260084.

Early E, Devine P. Why have a men's health policy? [Internet]. Queen's University Belfast; 2020. Available from: http://qpol.qub.ac.uk/why-have-a-mens-health-policy/.

Goodyear V, Quennerstedt M. #Gymlad — young boys learning processes and health-related social media. Qual Res Sport Exerc Health. 2019; 12(1):18–33.

Grace B, Shawe J, Johnson S, Stephenson J. You did not turn up… I did not realise I was invited…: understanding male attitudes towards engagement in fertility and reproductive health discussions. Hum Reprod Open. 2019 Jun 17;2019(3):hoz014.

Hamilton M, Pacey A, Tomlinson M, Brison D, Shaw L, Turner C, Witjens L, Morris P, Brown C, Montuschi O, Adams J, Lieberman B, Speirs J. Working Party on sperm donation services in the UK: Report and recommendations. Hum Fertil (Camb). 2008;11(3):147–58.

Hammarberg K, Collins V, Holden C, Young K, McLachlan R. Men's knowledge, attitudes and behaviours relating to fertility. Hum Reprod Update. 2017;23(4):458–80.

Harlow AF, Zheng A, Nordberg J, Hatch EE, Ransbotham S, Wise LA. A qualitative study of factors influencing male participation in fertility research. Reprod Health. 2020;17(1):186.

Hashiloni-Dolev Y, Kaplan A, Rasmussen CAW, Kroløkke C. Gamete preservation: Knowledge, concerns and intentions of Israeli and Danish students regarding egg and sperm freezing. Reprod Biomed Online. 2020;41(5):957–65.

Hviid Malling GM, Pitsillos T, Tydén T, Hammarberg K, Ziebe S, Friberg B, Schmidt L. 'Doing it in the right order': Childless men's intentions regarding family formation. Hum Fertil (Camb). 2022;22:1–9.

Inhorn MC, Birenbaum-Carmeli D, Birger J, Westphal LM, Doyle J, Gleicher N, Meirow D, Dirnfeld M, Seidman D, Kahane A, Patrizio P. Elective egg freezing and its underlying socio-demography: A binational analysis with global implications. Reprod Biol Endocrinol. 2018;16(1):70.

Inhorn MC, Birenbaum-Carmeli D, Patrizio P. Elective egg freezing and male support: A qualitative study of men's roles in women's fertility preservation. Hum Fertil (Camb). 2020;10:1–8.

Kato T. Associations of gender role attitudes with fertility intentions: A Japanese population-based study on single men and women of reproductive ages. Sex Reprod Healthc. 2018;16:15–22.

Lewis EI, Missmer SA, Farland LV, Ginsburg ES. Public support in the United States for elective oocyte cryopreservation. Fertil Steril. 2016;106(5):1183–9.

Meissner C, Schippert C, von Versen-Höynck F. Awareness, knowledge, and perceptions of infertility, fertility assessment, and assisted reproductive technologies in the era of oocyte freezing among female and male university students. J Assist Reprod Genet. 2016;33(6):719–29.

Mogilevkina I, Stern J, Melnik D, Getsko E, Tydén T. Ukrainian medical students' attitudes to parenthood and knowledge of fertility. Eur J Contracept Reprod Health Care. 2016;21(2):189–94.

Nasab S, Shah JS, Nurudeen K, Jooya ND, Abdallah ME, Sibai BM. Physicians' attitudes towards using elective oocyte cryopreservation to accommodate the demands of their career. J Assist Reprod Genet. 2019;36(9):1935–47.

Pacey AA, Eiser C. Banking sperm is only the first of many decisions for men: what healthcare professionals and men need to know. Hum Fertil (Camb). 2011;14(4):208–17.

Pacey AA, Martins da Silva S. The effect of age on male fertility and the health of offspring. In: Aitken J, Mortimer D, Kovacs G, editors. Male and sperm factors that maximise IVF success. Cambridge University Press; 2020.

Pacey AA. Sperm donor recruitment in the UK. Obstet Gynaecol. 2010; 12:43–8.

Pennings G, Couture V, Ombelet W. Social sperm freezing. Hum Reprod. 2021;36(4):833–9.

Perloff WH, Steinberger E, Sherman JK. Conception with human spermatozoa frozen by nitrogen vapor technic. Fertil Steril. 1964;25: 501–4.

Sherman JK, Bunge RG. Observations on preservation of human spermatozoa at low temperatures. Proc Soc Exp Biol Med. 1953 Apr;82(4):686–8.

Smith KR. Paternal age bioethics. J Med Ethics. 2015;41(9):775–9.

Stewart TM, Liu DY, Garrett C, Brown EH, Baker HW. Recruitment bias in studies of semen and other factors affecting pregnancy rates in fertile men. Hum Reprod. 2009;24(10):2401–8.

Yu L, Peterson B, Inhorn MC, Boehm JK, Patrizio P. Knowledge, attitudes, and intentions toward fertility awareness and oocyte cryopreservation among obstetrics and gynecology resident physicians. Hum Reprod. 2016;31(2):403–11.

Index

altruistic, 191
American, xi, xiii, xv, xvi, 25, 38,
  68, 167, 168, 170–173,
  175–177, 181–183, 208, 215
andrology, xviii, 68, 222
anti-Müllerian hormone (AMH),
  109–119, 212, 213
antral follicle count (AFC),
  109–112
assisted reproductive technology
  (ART), 67, 78, 191, 193, 195

barriers, 90, 187, 190, 196, 197
bioethics, xvii, 68, 188
birth weight, 82

cancer patients, 33, 44, 74, 102,
  115, 117–119, 126, 127, 134,
  141, 143, 225, 229
controlled ovarian stimulation
  (COS), 124, 125, 127, 128, 130,
  136, 137

cryopreservation, vi, xiii, 16–26,
  32–34, 36–38, 41, 43, 44,
  47–49, 52, 53, 66–69, 71–81,
  83, 84, 87, 88, 100, 101,
  119, 123–125, 127, 134, 135,
  139, 155, 158, 159, 163, 164,
  167, 170, 206, 207, 221–223,
  225–233

deferred motherhood, xvi, 11–13,
  15, 32, 49, 87–91, 100,
  105, 168, 170, 180–182,
  193, 194
demographic, 5, 79, 86, 97, 171,
  172, 196, 197

education, xv, 6–8, 12–15, 67,
  70, 72, 84, 93, 98–100, 103,
  170, 172, 177, 222–224, 227,
  232
endometrial preparation, 82,
  143–145, 147

estradiol, 109, 110, 128, 131, 133, 134, 141, 143, 144, 147

family size, 7, 13, 44, 93
fertility preservation (FP), vi, xii, 26, 49, 50, 52, 53, 55–61, 67, 70, 74, 77, 102, 109, 113, 114–116, 123–125, 127–129, 131–143, 191, 197–199, 222, 225, 227, 228, 230, 232
fertility rates, 2, 5–8, 72, 73, 76, 77, 97, 98, 105
follicle-stimulating hormone (FSH), 59, 108–111, 113, 129, 134, 136, 138, 145

history, vi, 16–18, 23, 26, 45, 70, 87, 88, 116, 134, 172, 212, 213
housing, 8, 90, 92–94, 97

inducement, 191
interview, 171, 172, 225
in vitro fertilisation (IVF), 33, 36–38, 44, 48, 49, 55, 56, 68, 70–74, 76–79, 87, 100, 111–113, 126, 135, 141, 143, 154, 157–160, 162, 163, 167, 170, 171, 173–175, 193, 201, 206, 207, 209, 212, 226, 227
in vitro maturation (IVM), 56–59

male, 37, 87, 89, 91, 99, 104, 108, 132, 134, 139, 158, 170, 182, 206, 210, 213, 222–225, 227–233

masculinity, 231
maternal outcomes, 79, 81, 145
men, 8, 73, 87, 91, 94, 99, 101, 103, 104, 131–135, 172, 179, 181, 182, 222–233

neonatal outcomes, 74, 78–80, 82, 83, 139, 154, 215

oocyte donation, 73, 123, 147, 155, 159, 163, 164, 206, 209, 213
oocyte freezing, 32, 33, 35–38, 44, 45, 56, 70, 73, 74, 78, 107, 114, 123, 228
ovarian cortex, vi, 47, 52, 54, 70, 133
ovarian reserve test, 69, 109, 110–112, 114, 115

public funding, 187, 189, 193, 194, 201
public perceptions, 166–168

sex ratio, 8–10
slow freezing, 18–20, 22, 24, 36, 38–41, 68, 206
'social' egg freezing, ix, 87, 89, 91, 99, 102, 104
sperm, xviii, 17, 20, 32, 33, 35–38, 43, 70, 87, 88, 92, 104, 108, 126, 152, 154, 156–158, 163, 175, 181, 206, 208, 210, 213, 222, 223, 225–227, 230

systematic review, 80, 82, 128, 140, 144, 145, 153, 212, 214

transfer protocol, 122, 142, 144, 145

United Kingdom (UK), v, ix, xi, xii–xv, xviii, 12, 24, 25, 86–90, 92–98, 104, 105, 108, 116, 174, 183, 206, 210, 212, 213, 231

vitrification, v–vii, 19, 20, 22–24, 33, 39–44, 49, 50, 55, 57, 62, 68, 73, 74, 88, 100, 101, 123, 134, 136, 143, 167, 206–208, 210, 211, 213–215